READ IT BEFORE YOU

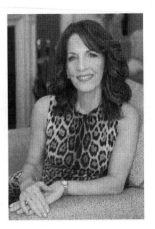

BONNIE TAUB-DIX, MA, RDN, CDN is the award-winning author of, *Read It Before You Eat It*, and creator of the website and blog called, *BetterThanDieting.com*. Bonnie is a **media personality, spokesperson, media trainer, motivational speaker, nutrition influencer, journalist,** and **corporate and brand consultant** whose messages are laced with her culinary passion, her credible guidance as an advisor and her wit and wisdom as a mom. Bonnie is Director and Owner of BTD Nutrition Consultants, LLC, with offices on Long Island and in New York City.

Her Master Course: *How to Work with the Media and Make the Media Work for You* is the only course you'll need if you want to get *your* name in the news and boost your media presence.

She has decades of extensive media experience (broadcast, online, print, social), where she has shared her expertise through outlets including: *TODAY* Show, *Martha Stewart Radio, New York Times, Washington Post, USA Today, US News & World Report* and a vast range of magazines and websites.

Her favorite pastime is cooking in the kitchen with her family. Even more important than some subjects you learn in school… Bonnie has set an example when setting her table by teaching her kids that nutritious and delicious can exist on the same plate.

On a personal note, Bonnie is grateful to be able to do what she loves every day and she takes pride in being referred to as, "genuine," "sincere," "reliable," and "professional." She is married and has three sons, a daughter-in-law and two grandchildren…all appreciators of good food!

What Bonnie brings to the plate –

Corporate Consultant & Advisory Board Member:

As Nutrition Communications Consultant to brands and corporate clients, Bonnie sees herself as being an interpreter, making sense of confusing science by helping to convey messages to consumers, industry, dietitians and health professionals via webinars, workshops, writing, and social media campaigns.

As a nutrition consultant to *The Cartoon Network*, Bonnie collaborated on designing a program for the Food and Drug Administration regarding food labeling, and to date, consults with CN on issues regarding programming and advertising to children.

As a liaison between industry and the public, she holds a position as an expert reviewer for *Livestrong.com* and *Greatist* to help assure that nutrition messages are clear, truthful and transparent.

Spokesperson:

Bonnie helps brands communicate and connect with their consumers by helping to craft realistic and meaningful campaigns that people can actually understand and apply to their everyday lives. Bonnie served as a Media Spokesperson to the New York State Dietetic Association for five years after which she was appointed to the position of Spokesperson for the Academy of Nutrition and

Dietetics for six years. She has conducted *thousands* of interviews for all forms of media and is called upon regularly as a trusted resource for television, magazines, newspapers, and web venues.

Television:
Bonnie has been a guest on national television shows including *CNN, CBS Early Show, ABC's Good Morning America, TODAY Show, Anderson Cooper 360, The Daily,* and *FOXNews.* She's worked with the *Discovery Channel* and *Lifetime TV* as an on-air consultant for several nationally broadcast programs. She is a contributor to TODAY.com.

Radio:
Bonnie has conducted Radio Media Tours and has been heard on many radio show including *Dr. Radio* on Sirius Satellite Radio and *Martha Stewart Radio.*

Print:
Bonnie published the first edition of her book, *Read It Before You Eat It*, translating confusing and misleading terminology into consumer-friendly information. Her strong relationships with members of the media have enabled her as a Registered Dietitian Nutritionist to guide shoppers down the supermarket aisle. Her book has been welcomed as a go-to resource in the food-labeling arena and has attracted hundreds of interviews in all forms of media. The evergreen and seemingly ever-confusing subjects of healthy supermarket shopping and label reading continue to be sited regularly.

Bonnie is a prolific writer on issues related to nutrition for both popular and professional publications providing practical advice on healthy living to the press including interviews via *New York Times, Washington Post, USA Today, The Daily News, The New York Post* and *The Chicago Tribune.* For two and a half years, she wrote a column for *Newsday*, and her articles and interviews have also appeared in magazines such as *Everyday with Rachel Ray, Health, Vogue, Shape, Fitness, Reader's Digest, Weight Watchers, Martha Stewart's Everyday Food, Ladies' Home Journal, Prevention, Women's Day,* and *Men's Health,* just to name a few.
She was a consultant to and quoted within books including *Nutrition for Dummies, Cholesterol for Dummies,* and *The Only 127 Things You Need*, and she has written chapters for textbooks, including *Weight Management: A Practical Guide, The Entrepreneurial Nutritionist,* and *Nutrition Concerns of Women.*

Bonnie is the co-author of *Kosher By Design Lightens Up*, a book that blends the science of nutrition and tradition of home cooking. Bonnie's cooking skills has helped to demonstrate that you can preserve tradition while preserving your health…all on the same plate.

Web:
Bonnie is a Contributor to *US News & World Report, TODAY.com, Better Homes & Gardens, What's Good V* (Vitamin Shoppe Blog), *Thrive Global,* and she had her own column, *Nutrition Intuition,* on *EverydayHealth*, writing about the hottest topics pertaining to diet and fitness. She wrote a weekly blog for *USA Today* for more than three years. Her storytelling draws much attention and her pieces are often reposted by other media and social media platforms such as *Huffington Post.* She has also guest blogged for sites that belong to corporate clients and other associations including International Food Information Council (IFIC).

Her quotes consistently appear on countless websites of national magazines and television shows.

Social Media Strategist:
Bonnie enjoys (and is a little obsessed with) connecting with her followers on social media. Bonnie particularly enjoys her role as a chat host in helping her corporate clients improve/enhance engagement on their social media platforms through Facebook LIVE videos, Twitter chats and Instagram takeovers. Her monthly twitter chats for Everyday Health brought more than 45 million impressions during a given chat. She has hosted chats for prominent clients including Starbucks, Nestle Waters of North America, and Grocery Manufacturers Association.

Culinary Skills:
Bonnie takes pride in creating recipes accompanied by her mouth-watering photographs shared in her stories and social media platforms, shining a light on her love for the beauty of food.

She is a #Foodiechats Ambassador, participating in twitter chats that draw millions of impressions each week.

With a great passion for and understanding of food science, she displays her creativity in developing recipes for brands and food companies and designing menus for restaurants.

Awards:
Bonnie has been honored with the 2012 Media Excellence Award by the Academy of Nutrition and Dietetics. In 2003, she received the Outstanding Nutrition Entrepreneur of the Year Award by the American Dietetic Association, and the following year she was acknowledged with the New York State Dietetic Association's Media Excellence Award.

Education:
Bonnie received her Bachelors Degree in Clinical and Community Dietetics from Downstate Medical Center and her Masters Degree in Nutrition from New York University.

Website: www.BetterThanDieting.com
Twitter: @eatsmartbd
Facebook: http://facebook.com/BonnieTaubDix.RDN
Instagram: @Bonnietaubdix and @BTDmedia
Pinterest: http://pinterest.com/bonnietaubdix/
Weekly News Digest: bit.ly/fCeEuT

Read It Before You Eat It

Taking You from Label to Table

Bonnie Taub-Dix, MA, RD, CDN

This book is dedicated to the four most amazing men in my life:
My husband, Mitch, for sharing his life with me, for always being there with sage and heartfelt advice, and for loving everything I cook (even when I'm just roasting garlic!)
And our three sons, Adam, Sam, and Jesse, who forever inspire me, teach me, and show me how they took my lead by shopping for, cooking with, and of course, enjoying the pleasure of delicious food.   I love and appreciate you all more than any words can ever express.

CONTENTS

Part Two

Navigating the Aisles: How to Shop for the Best Foods

ACKNOWLEDGMENTS

My heartfelt thanks go to all of those who helped me bring this book into being.

Credit goes to the countless patients who complained to me about how confusing food labels are and who trusted me to help them shop. Since I couldn't go to the store with each and every one of them … this book will sub as the closest thing to a personalized walk down the aisles.

To all of the public relations firms and brands I have collaborated with for years to help food companies create foods and messages that consumers could enjoy and benefit from.

To my assistant, Chelsey Amer, for her enthusiasm over helping me edit and update this book and for already being a shining light in our awesome profession.

To my dear family members and friends who put up with my book talk every step of the way and who show their love, interest, and support in my many nutrition-related ventures (especially my creations at family dinners).

A warm hug goes to my mom, Ruth Taub. Even though she is no longer with me, I'll never forget how she carried around a copy of my book in her purse to show everyone. She set an example through her unconditional love and perpetual optimism, and she taught me the meaning of empathy.

My most profound gratitude goes to my incredible husband Mitch, and my three extraordinary sons, Adam, Sam, and Jesse. Thank you so much for understanding why writing stood in the way of some creative cooking and baking. . . . I'm ready to take your requests now. And to my daughter-in-law Lindsay, for being an amazing listener and trend-watcher. I deeply appreciate all your support, enthusiasm throughout the days and sleepless nights I wrote this book and even more, throughout the days of our lives together. You have all grown to be my dearest BFFs; I am thankful every day to have a spouse and children that appreciate and understand all that I do. Thanks for being so willing to always voice your opinions (even if it seems like I don't really want to hear them!) and share your heartfelt thoughts. And big hugs to my new little grandson, Dylan, who I can't wait to cook with. Oh, and thanks to my dog Webster, who sat by my side till the wee hours of the morning while I typed away.

Each and every day, I truly appreciate the work I do and the people I do it with — and to those who are reading this book, thank you for letting me share my opinions with you. I am hoping you will pass what you've learned onto those you care about.

FOREWORD

When you enter a grocery store, you bring a lifetime of stored marketing messages with you that will influence your buying decisions, from advertising that has raised your awareness of product features to information that you have gotten from the Internet to your best friend's recommendation for her favorite brand.

Recently, we've also seen dozens of new terms — from "trans fat free" to "good source of antioxidants"— on our labels, and new nutritional ratings on shelves that can add to the confusion about what to buy. We didn't get to be a nation riddled with diabetes, clogged arteries, and heart disease by making smart eating decisions. We got this way because taste, price, and dozens of other marketing messages — rather than nutrition — have been foremost in our purchase decisions at the shelf.

When you're trying to shop healthfully for yourself and your family, it's important that you take responsibility for learning what you can from food labels and what they *really* mean, so the choices you make will be fully informed.

There is much more at stake here then the competitiveness of food brands and the retailers that sell them. Reading labels — and understanding them — has the potential to be a catalyst for a momentous turning point in the nation's health and wellness. In *Read It Before You Eat It*, Bonnie Taub-Dix is the teacher we have been searching for all these years. And now we need her more than ever before.

As we learn to read food labels and understand where our foods come from, how they are produced, and what's in them, we will retrain our taste buds and eating habits and we will be on the path to a much healthier way of eating, and with smiles on our faces.

You've taken the first step by deciding to read it *Read It Before You Eat It*. Now it's time to follow Bonnie as she takes us all on a remarkable journey that can change the way we eat forever.

Phil Lempert
Editor, SupermarketGuru.com and *The Lempert Report*
Contributor, *Today Show* and *The View*

INTRODUCTION

Why You Need This Supermarket Shopping Companion

Trying to lose weight, control diabetes, stabilize blood pressure, gain energy, or take control of your health through your diet? Chances are, you've tried all the latest crazes, from cleansing to carb-free, with little impact on your health. It can be incredibly frustrating to embark on diet after diet—each heralded as the magic formula to keep yourself thin and healthy—only to see meager results. Fortunately, there seems to be a shift in our culture toward a growing awareness of what we eat. People like Michael Pollan and Alice Waters encourage us to eat healthy whole foods and a diet composed mostly of fresh fruits and vegetables. As a dietitian nutritionist, I love this approach, but I also recognize that most of us face real-world constraints on our diets. Sure, it would be great to go to the farmers' market every day to pick up a freshly baked loaf of wholegrain bread, but realistically speaking, it's more likely that I'll swing by the grocery store for a loaf of a packaged pre-sliced type of bread. Once I'm there, I'll confront a shelf full of breads with packages that make all kinds of claims about how healthy they are, but how do you know which one will be best for you and your family? This book is meant to help you determine the best foods to buy by enlisting the aid of a powerful weapon that can help you succeed in your personal battle of the bulge and while trying to cut through the confusion— and that's the food label.

The label has been there for years, right in front of you, but you probably ignore it, don't you? I understand. And believe me, you're not alone. Labels can be misleading, full of terms you don't know (what is furcellaran anyway?) and hard to decipher. (FYI—furcellaran is an edible gum that is used to thicken foods.)

I want you to become a label reading expert. Learning to read labels and understand the numbers on your food package could help you to lose weight and gain control of the health issues that trouble you today, while preventing problems that may creep up on you tomorrow. You'll be able to make better, healthier decisions when shopping and cooking for you and your family. I'll help you to understand the difference between "sugar-free" and "no added sugar" and to determine whether it's better to buy "light" olive oil (spoiler: it's not!). I will walk you down the grocery store aisles and show you how to pick and choose the best foods out there no matter what your wallet holds or your taste buds desire.

The label is supposed to be like a table of contents of a book: It should describe what's contained inside. Typically, however, the front of a package looks more like a billboard, carrying advertisements designed to catch the eye of the hungry consumer. Some attention-grabbing packages seem to promise that their product is the answer to your aliments, curing everything from baldness to belly fat.

You might think that since labels are carefully regulated there would be no room for negotiation or misinterpretation about what goes on the package . . . right? Wrong. Labels are not just about government regulations and definitions, they are about educating and enticing consumers. But there are certain circumstances where the facts get twisted and some additional interpretation is necessary.

Some manufacturers till try to get away with using items like molasses, fruit juice concentrate, or honey, instead of table sugar, creating an illusion of a food substance that is healthy when, in fact, it provides lots of sweetness and empty calories from ingredients that may be just as sweet, but just may not be spelled, S-U-G-A-R. There might not be a grain of sugar, per se, in there, but these ingredients act like sugar when swallowed! "Fat-free" products are also repeat offenders. Don't be fooled into thinking fat-free means calorie-free. In fact, when it's a fat-free sweet treat like ice cream, it likely means it's laden with sugar. There are many food marketing tricks, such as listing small, unrealistic portion sizes to make a product seem low in calories, or using a word like "light" when the food is actually high in fat, sugar, salt, or calories. And when was the last time you checked the ingredient list? Not all strange-sounding items are harmful, but not all healthysounding ingredients are healthy either. Including these ingredients is often an attempt to make a product look more attractive or healthy, but it won't necessarily make you look more attractive or healthy.

And as long as you're reading my book, you might as well get to know me. I received a bachelor of science degree in Clinical and Community Dietetics from Downstate Medical Center and a master's in Nutrition from New York University. I am an award-winning author and creator of the website and blog called, BetterThanDieting.com. As a media personality, spokesperson, motivational speaker, nutrition influencer, journalist, and corporate and brand consultant my messages are laced with my culinary passion as a foodie, my credible guidance as an advisor and my wit and wisdom if I must say so myself!) as a mom. I am the Director and Owner of BTD Nutrition Consultants, LLC, with offices on Long Island and in New York City.

I take pride in my extensive media experience (broadcast, online, print, social), where I have shared my expertise through outlets including: TODAY Show, Martha Stewart Radio, New York Times, Washington Post, USA Today and a vast range of magazines and websites. I provide practical advice on healthy living and I consider it my mission to convert nutrition science into common sense, cutting through the often-conflicting medical studies and the shifting trends in dieting.

With all of this under my belt, so to speak, my favorite pastime is cooking in the kitchen with my family. Even more important than some subjects you learn in school...I have tried to set an example when setting my table by teaching my kids that nutritious and delicious can exist on the same plate.

On a personal note, I have been married for a very (ha!) very long time and I'm a mother of three incredible sons, a daughter-in-law and I have a new, adorable grandson. As the gatekeeper of meals and as a nutrition counselor, I've always tried to be realistic when teaching about choosing foods, while at the same time keeping in mind the individual's taste preference and state of health, always emphasizing that most foods can fit into a healthy diet.

I try to guide people by helping them to think of food in a different light: Each bite they eat will have a purpose and appear somewhere in their bodies. Whether it's to repair cells and tissues, give energy, or expand a waistline, the foods we eat have a variety of functions. For some, the key to making wise choices involves planning. I always liked the expression, "If you fail to plan, then you plan to fail." In my opinion, it's not obsessive if at breakfast time you're thinking ahead to what you're going to be eating for lunch or deciding what you're cooking for dinner. By coordinating your meals, you can balance out your day and assure that you're not going to overdo anything or be missing out on key nutrients your body needs.

This book will teach you how to focus in on the items on labels that pertain to you personally, according to your individual needs.

I couldn't even count the number of times a patient said to me, "I wish I could take you food shopping with me." They want me to help them translate what's on the label and cut through the confusion so they can make a quick, healthy decision about the best foods to buy. The typical supermarket carries 45,000 items and the average person buys 61 items in a 26-minute grocery shopping trip (that's 26 seconds per item). No wonder it's difficult to make a choice about what to throw in that shopping cart.

Since I can't actually go to the store with you, I will walk with you up and down the aisles of your supermarket and help explain confusing statements and deceptive labels on some of the products you've been purchasing for years. You'll also learn about how to compose a healthy diet without spending hours cooking in the kitchen or days in the library learning about nutrition. Moreover, I'll enable you to become skilled at separating fact from fiction by uncovering some of the most popular food myths that are highlighted by media hype, geared toward selling sound bites instead of sound advice.

So, this is what makes my book stand out from the rest: unlike food activists that just tell you what to do because they say so, *Read It Before You Eat It* will give you the opportunity to shop with me, a registered dietitian nutritionist who will take your individual needs into consideration. I'm not going to tell you what to do just because I said so — I'm going to give you the tools to help you decide which foods are best based upon a combo of science and common sense.

I'm hoping that *Read It Before You Eat It* will not only help make food shopping a painless experience for you, but that it will also assist you in making smarter and safer food choices for yourself and for your whole family.

After reading this book, you may not read the label on every product you purchase, but I'll bet you will flip over more packages than you did before to look at all sides of the box, not just the flashy front of the package, knowing that if you decide to spend your hard-earned money on a food, there's got to be a good reason why you chose that particular item. I hope that *Read It Before You Eat It* will help you navigate the aisles efficiently, safely, and healthfully.

Thanks for letting me come shopping with you. I'd love for you to fill your cart with food you'll feel proud to take from their labels to your table!

Part One

The Meaning Behind the Words on the Label . . . and Why You Should Care

Chapter 1

The History of Labeling: Where We Began and Where We're Going

If you grew up before the 1970s, there's a good chance that the food you bought didn't even have a detailed food label on it. In contrast to a billboard-like package of today, the old box may have described what was in that package, but it certainly didn't tell you what was actually in the food you were eating.

It's hard to believe that the Nutrition Facts Panel that appears on the side or back of our food products didn't develop until the 1970s. But that doesn't mean that our government was not interested in monitoring our food supply prior to that point. Believe it or not, the first food regulatory law was proclaimed by the king of England in the early thirteenth century, called *the Assize of Bread*, prohibiting bakers from mixing ground peas and beans into bread dough. These days you'd have to pay extra for such a bread, and it probably would be labeled as "highfiber/highprotein/multigrain" bread! In 1862, President Abraham Lincoln had our interests in mind when he launched the Department of Agriculture and the Bureau of Chemistry, the predecessor of the Food and Drug Administration (FDA).

In 1962, the code of food standards for all nations, called the Codex Alimentarius, was developed by an international commission, and it had a great impact on the quality and safety of the world's food supply, upgrading standards for food manufacturing, processing, safety, and quality all over the world. Our present food labeling program started out as a voluntary program overseen by the Food and Drug Administration (FDA) and the U.S. Department of Agriculture (USDA) in 1974. By the 1980s, there was a surge of interest in the field of nutrition and dietetics. Around that time, the Surgeon General of the U.S. Public Health Service and the National Academy of Sciences' National Research Council released two reports, entitled the "Surgeon General's Report on Nutrition and Health" (1988) and the "National Research Council's Diet and Health: Implications for Reducing Chronic Disease Risk" (1989). These papers concluded that there was a strong association between diet and risk of chronic disease, which then lead to recommendations for dietary changes and the need for a revised food label.

Registered dietitian nutritionists and public health experts recommended that Americans lose weight, lower their cholesterol, saturated fat, sugar and sodium levels, and increase the amounts of calcium and fiber they consumed. Doesn't that sound familiar? I just saw an article yesterday that made the same suggestions.

Consumers literally ate up the new products that were hitting the shelves along with the promises they brought with them. Manufacturers responded in kind to consumer interest regarding the connection between food and its effect on disease prevention, and health claims appeared everywhere. If a claim was made about a particular item, say, "low in fat," a more detailed label was required, but labels were not as specific as they are today.

Consumer interest groups expressed concern regarding the potential for harm if manufacturers conveyed false or misleading messages to the public and, in response, Congress passed the Nutrition Labeling and Education Act (NLEA) in 1990 as an amendment to the existing 1938 Federal Food,

Drug, and Cosmetic Act. The NLEA gave the FDA the authority to protect consumers by developing regulations requiring that packaged food contain labels carrying information regarding their nutrient levels. This was in part formulated with the hope that manufacturers would create healthier foods in accordance with the current scientific studies encouraging the consumption of foods lower in fat, cholesterol, sodium, and sugar. The legislation led to more truth in labeling and the availability of a greater wealth of information for consumers. But did this information lead to better food choices? To this day we're still trying to get manufacturers to produce, and consumers to choose, foods that contain less of the same four diet offenders. It's hard to believe that even with this country's rich food supply, and with nutrition information bombarding us regularly on television and radio, in web sites, social media, and magazines and newspapers, that studies still show that adults and children are not getting enough of the valuable nutrients they need on a daily basis (such as fiber, calcium, iron, and vitamins A, C and D). Conversely, with the majority of our adult population either overweight or obese, overdosing on other nutrients (total fat, saturated fat, cholesterol, sugar, and sodium) does not mean that we are well fed.

After counseling hundreds of patients who have been frustrated by the ambiguous statements on food packages, I hope to teach you how to make quick, valuable decisions when faced with that box, bag, or bottle before you make your purchase. And, through my simple guidelines, you can become skilled at setting an example for your children, leading them to make smarter, more independent food choices. Learning how to read a label is an important lesson from which you and your family will reap a lifetime of benefits.

From Your Heart to Your Cart: Why Do We Choose the Foods We Choose?

Why did you choose the food you ate today? Let's take a look at your breakfast: Did you scramble up some eggs, put a slice or two of whole-grain bread in the toaster, and brew a steamy mug of tea to give you a nice warm start to your day? Or did your morning begin with grabbing a muffin or donut and a cup of coffee at a local coffee shop on the way to your office? Perhaps you shoved down a few bites of the breakfast and/or lunch you made for your kids while standing at the counter in your kitchen before running off to drive for the carpool. Maybe you skipped breakfast altogether.

Whatever your reason (or excuse) was, you actually had to think about what you were going to do before making that breakfast choice. Dr. Brian Wansink, the director of the Cornell University Food and Brand Lab in New York, has shown in his research that the average person makes well over two hundred decisions about food every day. In his book *Mindless Eating*, Wansink shows how we can eliminate some of the "hidden persuaders," as he calls them, which lead us to overeat. We often have good intentions about curbing our intake…until temptation takes over—whether it's jelly beans in a glass jar on your countertop or free samples at the supermarket. Supermarkets are set up in the way they want you to shop. By placing an appealing item at the entrance of the store, like freshly cut flowers or freshly baked loaves of bread, we are drawn to buying those products.

That's why 60 to 70 percent of what ends up in our shopping carts is unplanned.

Sometimes we really don't have a choice about what we eat. If you're at an all-day meeting that includes a lunch, or if you're a dinner guest at a friend's house, you may not have much of a say when it comes to the food du jour. In these situations, you may feel like a captive audience. There are other times, however, when you may blame poor food decisions on the fight you had with your husband or the kids who made you crazy or the boss who didn't give you a raise, but in reality, the person who made you dig your fork into that food and lift it to your lips was none other than you.

We each select food for different reasons: whether it's our culture and upbringing, our friends, family and coworkers, religious beliefs, or our budget and environment, there are a variety of factors that dictate what we eat and why.

It's All in a Name

When products are given descriptive names, such as "freshly baked," "homemade," "natural," or "wholesome," they appear more attractive. Restaurants are well aware of this phenomenon. Dr. Wansink has shown on numerous occasions that certain glasses, plates, and menu descriptions can unknowingly cause us to eat too much. He found that when descriptive names (*Black Forest Double-Chocolate Cake* as opposed to *Chocolate Cake*) were used on menus, people would rate the foods as tasting better. Further results showed that descriptive menu labels (such as Grandma's Zucchini Cookies or Succulent Italian Seafood Fillet increased sales by 27 percent and improved attitudes toward the food, attitudes toward the restaurant, and a greater likelihood of coming back to the restaurant. They even indicated that they would be willing to pay almost 10 percent more for each descriptive menu item. This highlighted how easily people are influenced simply by labels. Making foods more alluring via descriptive names is not limited to restaurants. Manufacturers love to attract shoppers in supermarkets with eye-catching displays, fancy packaging, and striking names for basic foods.

Numerous studies have concluded that the most effective way to lose weight is by eating less. No surprise there. This simple theory that I have been teaching patients for more than thirty five years is not as simple as it sounds. Modifying your diet takes a tremendous amount of patience, tolerance, understanding, and education. Reports even show that men shop for food differently than women do. Women are often found to have more trouble suppressing their appetites, making sex— along with friends—one more factor in what they choose to eat.

There are dozens of reasons why we choose the foods we do—from your family history, or who you're friends with, or even whether you had a bad day at work. The fact is that more than two-thirds of the population in United States is overweight or obese. Media stories cite genetics as one culprit in this crisis, pointing to your parents, grandparents, and distant relatives as the reasons why your pants don't zip up. Although many studies have shown that your genes play an important role in whether your jeans fit, other research has shown that your life at home (your environment) also has a significant effect on what you're putting in your grocery cart.

It is also said that people tend to align themselves with people who resemble them, and having overweight friends may change your idea about which body weight is socially acceptable, so that the more overweight the people are within your social network, the more likely you are to accept being heavy.

Obesity rates have risen among all socioeconomic groups, spreading within social networks and from person to person. Now I'm not saying that you can "catch" obesity like you can catch the common cold, but perhaps you are more influenced by others than you realize about whether to have fries or a salad with your sandwich. External influences can be powerful, and they can work for or against you.

I'm not suggesting that you choose your partner, friends, or social contacts in accordance with their eating style or by their body size, but if you're trying to watch your weight, it may help to become more aware of how the people in your life affect the choices you make at the table. Stick to your guns: Choose food because you need it (you're hungry) or because you want it (perhaps caloric but worthwhile). If you're dining in a restaurant, try to think about what will be on the menu ahead of time, and if you're going food shopping, be sure to bring your list with you and don't go hungry. Don't eat because of anyone else, because no one else wears your clothes. Perhaps the bottom line is to listen to what your mother told you—choose your friends (and food) wisely.

Labels That Lure You

When it comes to what influences *your* personal food choices when food shopping, one of the biggest hidden persuaders is the food label.

A survey conducted by the International Food Information Council (IFIC) from March of 2007 found that consumers had what the researchers termed "diet disconnects." Seventy percent of Americans who said they are trying to improve the healthfulness of their diet reported they are doing so in order to lose weight. But only 11 percent of Americans knew the number of calories they should consume each day.

Shoppers seemed to be familiar with the list of basic nutrients like carbohydrates, calcium, and vitamin C and trendy food terms like omega-3 fatty acids and lycopene, but name recognition didn't mean that consumers understood how nutrients benefit the body, what foods they're found in, how much of a nutrient they are supposed to have in a day, or how this information applies to their lifestyles. It also seems that consumers became more myopic about paying attention to one component or another—like trans fats or sodium—if they heard a lot about it in the media.

When faced with food labels boasting "fat-free" or "sugar-free," consumers acted as if they received an invitation to indulge, leading to the consumption of portions sizes well beyond those needed. This is one of the most common mistakes people make. These terms on food labels are providing information to help consumers meet their dietary recommendations, particularly if they have special requirements, like needing to watch their cholesterol intake, but these words do not automatically mean that the food is calorie-free, or even calorie-reduced. For that guidance, you must check the calories and serving sizes listed on the Nutrition Facts Panel, and pay close attention to how many servings are contained within one package…which the new Nutrition Facts label is making even easier to discern.

From Guidelines to Your Grocery Cart

Learning how to interpret the truth and consequences regarding the terms and claims on food labels is just one piece of the puzzle. Let's start by facing the facts—the nutrition facts, that is, and we'll decipher what's appearing on your food label.

Chapter 2

Ready, Set, Shop: Gathering the Guidelines

Consumers often look for miracle foods that can provide everything they need in one nifty little package. That's like expecting one instrument to play the sounds of an entire symphony. No one food can give you everything you need. It takes a variety and a balance of nourishing foods to help you stay fit—both physically and emotionally.

When I try to explain the concept of *balancing* foods, I sometimes use the following illustration: If you were getting dressed and you put on a shirt, and then you put on a shirt and next you put on a shirt . . . you would not be dressed appropriately. You'd be wearing too many shirts and not enough of the other things you'd need to make your outfit complete (pants, socks, shoes, etc.). Similarly, when it comes to our diets, some of us wake up in the morning and have some sort of muffin, roll, bagel, or pastry. Then lunch becomes two quick slices of pizza and dinner may consist of a big bowl of pasta with sauce. While we did a great job of getting our fill of carbs, some other crucial items are missing—like protein, dairy, and other nutrients. Carbohydrates are not the bad guys, they are simply not *balanced* properly with other foods.

When putting together a healthy diet, you need a little bit of everything to make it work. Eating healthfully is not just about an individual food on a given day, it's about your total intake over the course of days, weeks, months, and years.

When I grew up in the 1960s, we learned about the "Basic Four" food groups: grains, meat, milk, and fruits and vegetables. Those four food groups, however, lacked depth; the system didn't differentiate between a piece of meat marbled with fat and a lean chicken breast, nor did it encourage skim rather than full-fat milk. The dietary recommendations encouraged well-rounded meals, and it probably was physical activity that kept Americans from looking more "wellrounded." In those days, kids played ball and rode bikes—rather than surf the web or get glued to a tablet or smartphone, they burned calories.

Next came the 70s, which brought concerns about getting more food than needed and preventing diseases of affluence like heart disease and obesity. The 1977 Dietary Goals for the United States expanded the Basic Four to include a fifth group – fats, sweets, and alcohol – which Americans were encouraged to limit.

Over time, several versions of goals and guidelines were established by our government, leading to the present-day *Dietary Guidelines for Americans* (which was most recently updated and upgraded in 2015). The purpose of these Guidelines is to provide a total diet approach of what we should be eating based on the most recent research. In the 1980s we followed the "Food Wheel," which was replaced by the Food Guide Pyramid in 1992, and updated in 2005 to MyPyramid, in an attempt to translate nutritional recommendations into the types and the amounts of food to eat each day.

The pyramid and its revisions were a good start, but lacked the clarity that Americans needed as an example to set the table nutritiously. In 2011, My Plate was introduced along with the *2010 Dietary Guidelines for Americans* to paint a clear picture of what the average plate should look like to provide well-balanced, nutritious meals. Using a realistic plate allowed consumers to visualize this reminder of healthy eating.

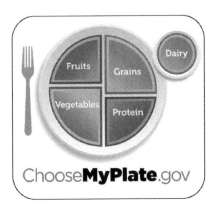

ChooseMyPlate.gov

If you log on to www.ChooseMyPlate.gov, you'll find a wealth of information for yourself and the whole family, including a guide that will tell you how much of each food group to choose each day, depending upon your age, height, weight, gender, and level of activity. ChooseMyPlate.gov provides a tool called SuperTracker, which allows you to enter your personal profile to obtain a detailed diet and menu plan without ever leaving your home and without costing you a penny. This platform allows you to set specific health goals, weight loss or maintenance goals, physical activity goals, along with a variety of tracking tools. The Food Tracker tool acts as an online food journal, comparing your intake to your personal goals. The Activity Tracker allows you to keep track of your physical activity. You can also opt in to receive email support through the "My Coach Center," to receive daily or weekly tips to help you achieve your goals. Here's a sample of what you might find:

Each guideline starts with a recommendation for daily calories. For example, a moderately active thirty-five-year-old woman is advised to aim for 2,200 calories a day. And how should she divvy these calories up to get everything she needs? Here's the advice:

- Fruits: 2 cups
- Vegetables: 3 cups
- Grains: 7 ounce equivalents (at least half of which should be whole grains)
- Protein foods: 6 ounce equivalents
- Dairy: 3 cups
- Oils: 6 teaspoons

The guidelines also point out other dietary components that she should limit: added sugars, saturated fat, and sodium.

The site provides links to a list of helpful tips, like a chart that explains the concept of a "cup of fruit." (A half cup of dried fruit counts as a cup. So does one large apple, two medium plums, eight large strawberries, and thirty-two seedless grapes.) If you're not sure what an "ounce equivalent" means, you'll find that both a slice of bread and ½ cup of cooked pasta each count as an "ounce equivalent" of grain. Likewise, one ounce of lean meat or poultry is equivalent to one egg or ½ ounce of nuts.

If you are new to planning your meals and the Dietary Guidelines, the vast quantity of information that is available may be overwhelming. For example, the guidelines break down the vegetables into five different categories. Our active thirty-five-year-old woman is told that her weekly diet should include 2 cups of dark green vegetables, 6 cups of red and orange vegetables, 2 cups of beans and legumes, 6 cups of starchy vegetables, and 5 cups of "other vegetables" (such as cucumbers, mushrooms, and cauliflower). But if you're a novice at attempting to follow a healthier eating plan, aiming to eat 3 cups of vegetables daily, regardless of *the color*, may be a more appropriate goal than worrying about if you're eating the "right" amount of orange vegetables. Then, as you progress through your healthy eating journey, you will continuously be able to set new goals for yourself through the help of the wealth of information provided on the MyPlate website.

Fast Fact

No fresh fruit? Try dried. A quarter cup of dried fruit counts as ½ cup fresh fruit, or one fruit serving.

What about those other dietary components: added sugars, saturated fat, and sodium? The 2015 Dietary Guidelines for Americans suggest limiting added sugars and saturated fat to less than 10% of calories per day and sodium intake to less than 2,300 milligrams (mg) per day. If you're not a mathematician, it may be difficult to understand all of these numbers! For a 2,200-calorie diet, limiting added sugars and saturated fat to 10% of total daily calories each would equal 220 calories or 55 grams of added sugar per day and 220 calories or 24 grams of saturated fat daily. One teaspoon of salt contains around 2,300 mg of sodium. Even if you have shaken the habit of throwing salt on your food before you taste it, most of the sodium we get in our diets come from highly processed and packaged foods, which is where reading food labels properly comes into play.

(See Chapter 3: Label Lingo for more information on finding hidden sources of sodium!)

An important point to make here is that the thirty-five-year-old woman used as our reference is active and not overweight. If she needed to lose weight, her caloric intake would be more limited than the plan that is outlined.

As discovered in numerous market research studies, including the 2016 Food and Health Survey conducted by the International Food and Information Council Foundation (IFIC), most people are trying to include more healthful foods – fruits, vegetables, whole grains, and plant based sources of protein -- into their diets, but this doesn't equate with really knowing what or how much they should be eating each day. Some research highlights that Americans are very likely to overestimate or underestimate their caloric intake, making it more difficult to choose the right foods in the proper amounts.

The Label Makeover

To help consumers make healthier food choices, in May 2016, the Food and Drug Administration (FDA) announced that the Nutrition Facts panel on the back of our food packages will be getting a major makeover. The updated Nutrition Facts panel aims to help consumers seamlessly make healthier food choices.

Dietary Reference Intakes (DRIs) consist of four reference values, based on age and gender: 1) Recommended Dietary Allowances (RDAs), 2) Estimated Average Requirement (EAR), 3)

Adequate Intake (AI), and 4) Tolerable Upper Level (UL). The DRI values are not currently used in nutrition labeling, but instead, the Daily Value (DV), or a single value for each nutrient that is needed, is used instead. Note that the DV is typically very close to the RDA or AI for a given nutrient.

The percent DV represents the amount thought to meet or exceed the requirements of practically all those within the population. It would be impossible to list the needs of each individual on a food label; a label cannot take into account whether you need to lose or gain weight or whether you are a marathon runner or armchair athlete. The DV on the Nutrition Facts panel has not been updated since the original food label in 1993, but the revised Nutrition Facts panel will reflect updated nutrient recommendations that have since been released.

The following is a guide you can use to help determine how much of certain important nutrients you need each day. This chart is based upon the updated nutrient recommendations that will be reflected in the percent Daily Value (%DV) on the new Nutrition Facts panel, for those four years or older, eating 2,000 calories per day.

Food Labeling Reference Tables

For those four years or older, eating 2,000 calories per day, the updated Daily Values are:

Total fat	78 grams
Saturated fat	20 grams
Cholesterol	300 mg
Sodium	2,300 mg
Potassium	4,700 mg
Total carbohydrate	275 grams
Fiber	28 grams
Protein	50 grams

For vitamins and minerals, the DRIs are given in the following table, along with the more recent RDAs of the Dietary Reference Intakes (maximized over sex and age groups)

Nutrient	DRI	Highest RDA of DRI
Vitamin A	3,000 IU	10,000 IU
Vitamin C	60 mg	90 mg
Calcium	1,300 mg	1,300 mg
Iron	18 mg	18 mg
Vitamin D	15 mcg	15 mcg
Nutrient	DRI	Highest RDA of DRI
Vitamin E	30 IU	15 mg (33 IU of synthetic)
Vitamin K	80 mcg	120 mcg
Thiamin	1.5 mg	1.2 mg
Riboflavin	1.7 mg	1.3 mg

Niacin	20 mg	16 mg
Vitamin B_6	2 mg	1.7 mg
Folate	400 mcg	400 mcg
Vitamin B_{12}	6 mcg	2.4 mcg
Biotin	300 mcg	30 mcg
Pantothenic acid	10 mg	5 mg
Phosphorus	1,000 mg	1,250 mg
Iodine	150 mcg	150 mcg
Magnesium	400 mg	420 mg
Zinc	15 mg	11 mg
Selenium	70 mcg	55 mcg
Copper	2 mg	900 mcg
Manganese	2 mg	2.3 mg
Chromium	120 mcg	35 mcg
Molybdenum	75 mcg	45 mcg
Chloride	3,400 mg	2,300 mg

The new food labeling system is designed to help us make better and quicker decisions, by highlighting calories, noting more realistic serving sizes, and pointing out added sugar. In the next chapter, we will dive in all the label lingo you need to know to be a supermarket sleuth!

To look more closely at your specific needs, you may want to consult a registered dietitian nutritionist or log on to www.ChooseMyPlate.gov.

Once you have a good idea of what kinds of foods you should be shopping for, how do you make sure you're choosing the right foods at the grocery store? Continue reading so you can decode what's on the label and make supermarket shopping a breeze instead of an overwhelming chore.

Chapter 3

Label Lingo

One of the most common questions I get asked by reporters, by the people who attend my workshops and by my patients is, "What's the most important item to look at on the label?" It's a good question, as there's so much information on food labels and these labels can be confusing and misleading. The answer to this question, however, is not so simple.

What do *you* look for when you turn your favorite food package over and check the Nutrition Facts Panel? Do you look at how many calories are packed into the box because you're trying to lose weight but don't necessarily care about where those calories coming from? Or do you check the label's fat and cholesterol content because your doctor just read you the riot act and threatened to put you on cholesterol-lowering medication? Or perhaps you have diabetes and you're trying to watch your intake of added sugar, but you've heard that it's also important to check the grams of carbohydrate, fiber, and sugar alcohols because each of these components could have an impact on blood glucose levels, too.

If you're confused, you're not alone.

What's on the Label?

According to the Nutrition Labeling and Education Act (NLEA), *all* packaged food products are required to contain the following information:

- Common name of the product
- Name and address of the product's manufacturer
- Net contents in terms of weight, measure, or count
- Ingredient list and Nutrition Facts Panel

The updated Nutrition Facts label, coming to packaged foods in your supermarket soon, will bring consumers:

- Nutrition information about almost every food in the grocery store
- Distinctive, improved, easy-to-read formats that enable consumers to find the information they need to make healthful food choices
- Information on the amount per serving of saturated fat, added sugars, dietary fiber, and other nutrients of major health concern
- Nutrient reference values, expressed as percent Daily Values, to help consumers see how a food fits into an overall daily diet
- Uniform definitions for terms that describe a food's nutrient content—such as "light," "lowfat," and "high-fiber"—to ensure that such terms mean the same for all products on which they appear
- Claims about the relationship between a nutrient or food and a disease or health-related condition, such as calcium and osteoporosis, and fat and cancer. These are helpful for people who are concerned about eating foods that may help keep them healthier longer.

16

- Standardized, more realistic serving sizes that make nutritional comparisons of similar products easier

The Nutrition Facts Panel: You Can't Afford to Skip It

All manufacturers were required to include a Nutrition Facts Panel on their products by 1994. (see figure 2). Although it has received a couple of facelifts since then (with the most recent makeover hitting store shelves by 2018), this label applies to packaged foods regulated by the FDA, but it does not apply to all food products. For example, the National Labeling and Education Act (NLEA) does not include meat and poultry products, because they are regulated by the U.S. Department of Agriculture (USDA).

Just imagine how challenging it is to present a food product label that is informative, unique, honest, and concise. NLEA guidelines also require that products have to be "within the context of the total daily diet," as well as measure up against similar products. In addition, manufacturers have taken advantage of the information listed on the Nutrition Facts Panel by highlighting certain items for their own benefit. Here's an example: When fat was thought to be a close relative of poison in the 1970s, manufacturers started making "fat-free" versions of some of their best sellers, particularly in the cookie aisle. Though a product, like "fat-free" cookies may have boasted that it's a "fat-free" food, if you flipped that package over, you'd notice that although the fat content may be low in comparison to comparable products, the sugar and calorie content may be higher than the original product made by the same company.

> **Where do *you* get your nutrition information?**
>
> According to the International Food Information Council's *2016 Food & Health Survey*, consumers claim that their top three trusted sources for guidance on the types of foods they should be eating are, respectively, Registered Dietitian Nutritionists, personal healthcare professionals, and the US government agencies, which has changed from seven years ago when the media, food labels, and family/friends were ranked as the top three sources of guidance for making food choices. Interestingly, the Nutrition Facts Panel (NFP) has declined in popularity as the primary thing that consumers look at on the label. Now, seven out of ten consumers consider the expiration date the most important piece of information on a food or beverage package.

The New Nutrition Facts Panel

As of January 2020, manufacturers must include the updated Nutrition Facts Panel on all packaged food products (smaller businesses have until the following year), however, you may already see the updated Panel on some packaged foods. Figure 2 below shows a side-by-side comparison of the current label (as of 2016) on the left and the updated label on the right.

Nutrition Facts

Serving Size 2/3 cup (55g)
Servings Per Container About 8

Amount Per Serving

Calories 230	Calories from Fat 72
	% Daily Value*
Total Fat 8g	**12%**
Saturated Fat 1g	**5%**
Trans Fat 0g	
Cholesterol 0mg	**0%**
Sodium 160mg	**7%**
Total Carbohydrate 37g	**12%**
Dietary Fiber 4g	**16%**
Sugars 1g	
Protein 3g	
Vitamin A	10%
Vitamin C	8%
Calcium	20%
Iron	45%

* Percent Daily Values are based on a 2,000 calorie diet. Your daily value may be higher or lower depending on your calorie needs.

	Calories:	2,000	2,500
Total Fat	Less than	65g	80g
Sat Fat	Less than	20g	25g
Cholesterol	Less than	300mg	300mg
Sodium	Less than	2,400mg	2,400mg
Total Carbohydrate		300g	375g
Dietary Fiber		25g	30g

Nutrition Facts

8 servings per container
Serving size   2/3 cup (55g)

Amount per serving

Calories   230

	% Daily Value*
Total Fat 8g	**10%**
Saturated Fat 1g	**5%**
Trans Fat 0g	
Cholesterol 0mg	**0%**
Sodium 160mg	**7%**
Total Carbohydrate 37g	**13%**
Dietary Fiber 4g	**14%**
Total Sugars 12g	
Includes 10g Added Sugars	**20%**
Protein 3g	
Vitamin D 2mcg	10%
Calcium 260mg	20%
Iron 8mg	45%
Potassium 235mg	6%

* The % Daily Value (DV) tells you how much a nutrient in a serving of food contributes to a daily diet. 2,000 calories a day is used for general nutrition advice.

Figure 2. Nutrition Facts Panel

There are several key changes to the Nutrition Facts Panel that manufactures are required to abide by. They are:

1. Serving Size and Servings per container

   Both the "Serving size" and the "servings per container" will now be in a larger font and/or bolder font to draw emphasis to these key pieces of information. Additionally, the updated label will feature more realistic serving sizes that closer reflect what people actually eat and drink. Finally, we may no longer see '1/5 of a bag' of microwave popcorn as a serving size when we all know that a bag like that can become a serving for one person when paired with a good TV show!

2. Calories

   Calories are one of the first pieces of information many consumers look at on a Nutrition Facts panel, which is why it will be larger and bolder on the new label.

3. Fats

   Fat phobia is finally coming to a close! The new Nutrition Facts Panel will no longer feature "Calories from Fat," as we know that not all fats are created equally! Some foods that contain fat, such as oil or nuts, actually benefit our health. Total Fat, Saturated Fat and Trans Fat will all still be required on food labels. *Did you ever pay attention to 'calories from fat' anyway?*

4. Added Sugars

   There is a big difference between natural sugar (the sugar within fruit and milk) and added sugar (the sugar added by the food company), and we're finally going to see the difference between the two as reflected on new food labels. Manufacturers are now required to report the quantity of "Added Sugars," in grams and as a percent Daily Value (%DV), on the Nutrition Facts label to comply with the updated 2015 Dietary Guidelines for Americans, which state that no more than 10% of total daily calories should come from added sugars. Research has shown that it is difficult to maintain a healthful diet if more than 10% of total daily calories come from added sugars.

5. Micronutrients

Only certain micronutrients (vitamins and minerals) are required to be included on the Nutrition Facts Panel. The new 2018 label will feature an updated list, with an actual amount in grams, in addition to the %DV to be listed. Vitamin D and potassium are now required on the label because so many Americans do not get the recommended amounts of those nutrients, which puts them at higher risk for chronic disease. Vitamins A and C are no longer required since deficiencies of these vitamins are rare today, however, these nutrients may still be included on a voluntary basis.

Based on newer scientific evidence, the daily values for some nutrients [including sodium, calcium and vitamin D] have also been updated.

6. Percent Daily Value (%DV)

If you've never noticed the footnote at the bottom of the Nutrition Facts Panel before, you certainly will now that I'm pointing it out! The footnote at the bottom of the label currently attempts to explain the meaning of %DV, but is more confusing than need be, and the FDA is hoping their re-wording helps to alleviate consumer confusion. Remember, the %DV helps you understand how a certain nutrient fits into the context of your total diet. On the Nutrition Facts label, the %DV is explained in terms of a 2,000 calorie per day diet.

In addition to the "Serving Size" and "Servings per container," manufacturers are required to provide information on specific nutrients on the Nutrition Facts label. The mandatory and voluntary nutrient components and the order in which they must appear are:

- total calories
- total fat
- saturated fat
- polyunsaturated fat
- monounsaturated fat
- cholesterol
- sodium
- total carbohydrate
- dietary fiber
- soluble fiber
- insoluble fiber
- total sugars
- added sugars
- sugar alcohols (for example, the sugar substitutes xylitol, mannitol, and sorbitol)
- protein
- vitamin D

- vitamin A
- percent of vitamin A present as beta-carotene
- vitamin C
- calcium
- iron
- potassium
- other essential vitamins and minerals [phosphorus, magnesium, vitamin K, vitamin B12, etc.]

If a claim is made about any of the optional or "voluntary" components, or if a food is fortified or enriched with any of them, nutrition information for these components becomes mandatory. These mandatory and voluntary components are the only ones allowed on the Nutrition Facts Panel. The nutrients were selected because they address today's public health concerns.

Let's take a look at these components…

Servings per Container

The number of servings per container tells you how many serving sizes are in the whole package. So if one serving is 1 cup, and the entire package has 5 cups, there are 5 servings per package. Many people skip this essential number, which is why the new label lists Servings per Container on the first line of the label.

When looking at the Nutrition Facts Panel, it's a good idea to compare the calories and nutrients and serving size with other products to help you make the best choice.

The Serving Size

The second row of information on the updated Nutrition Facts Panel is Serving Size. This amount is determined by the food manufacturer, but should reflect the amount that people generally eat. As stated above, what is now considered a single serving size is typically larger than what was considered a standard serving years ago; this shift will be reflected in the new Nutrition Facts label. All of the information about the nutritional value of the food that is listed on the label is given according to the serving size listed. So if a serving size is 2 crackers and you eat 8 crackers (or 4 servings), you need to quadruple all of the nutrition information on the label. All too often, this information is deceiving. For example, a packaged muffin may contain 300 calories per serving, but if the serving size listed on the label is "½ muffin," then there will be 2 servings per package and the actual muffin will contain 600 calories. I have not come across many people who would eat only half of a muffin and leave the rest for another day, which is why the updated serving size on the 2018 Nutrition Facts label should list this same muffin as 1 serving, containing 600 calories.

New Label Benefits!

Calories

The calorie section on the food table is like the star of a show. Our nation has an obsession with calories, but that doesn't mean that we know *where* our calories are coming from or *how* they contribute to what we look and feel like—we just know it's a number that's important. What is a calorie anyway?

A calorie is a unit of energy; it measures how much energy a food provides to the body. The number of calories listed on the food label indicates how many calories are in *one serving* of that particular food. If you're watching your weight, it's important to be mindful of the amount of calories you eat each day *and* to be aware of the *type* of calories you eat.

Calories come from both foods and beverages. If you're overweight, it's probably not just one nutrient causing the problem. For example, if a product is "fat-free," it may still contain a lot of calories coming from carbohydrates or sugar, and it may contain the same number of calories as a similar product that is not fat-free. Here's where "free" could be costly! Eating too many "diet" products could lead to excessive consumption of calories, which could turn into a recipe for obesity. If a food package says "low-something" on the label, it doesn't automatically mean that your calorie intake will be low. To trim your body, you have to trim your portion sizes.

Total Fat

Fat has gotten a bad rap over the years. We have been led to believe that if you eat fat, you'll get fat. The misconception is that *all* types of fat have a negative impact on health. The real problem with fat is that we eat too much of it.

The number of grams of fat listed on the Nutrition Facts Panel indicates how much fat is in a single serving of food. Although eating too much fat can lead to obesity and related health problems, our bodies do need some fat every day, and current research focuses on the *type* of fat we eat, rather than just the total amount consumed. Why do we need fat?

Fats are an important source of energy and, as a matter of fact, they contain twice as much energy per gram (9 calories) as carbohydrates or protein (4 calories each). While low-carb diets still enjoy some popularity, the reality is that carbohydrates contain less than half the calories of fat. High-carb foods that are also high in fat (muffins and cakes) are another story!

Fats have many important roles to play in the body:

- Fats provide insulation and cushioning for the skin, bones, and internal organs.
- Fat carries and helps store certain vitamins (A, D, E, and K) and hormones.
- Fat provides mouth-feel, satiety and satisfaction from foods, which can help us eat less.

Eating too much fat, however, can contribute to health problems, including heart disease and cancer.

The fats you eat should be liquid in nature, such as olive or canola oil, and rich in omega-3 fatty acids, in nuts and fish, instead of solid trans fats (in hydrogenated margarines) or saturated fats (in butter).

Fast Fact

When it comes to comparing the calories of the major nutrients, fats provide twice as many calories per gram (9 calories) as carbohydrates or protein (4 calories each). Alcohol provides 7 calories per gram, so watch out for liquid calories, too.

The Good, the Bad, and the Ugly: Unsaturated Fat, Saturated Fat, and Trans Fats

Paying attention to the Nutrition Facts Panel will help you know which types of fat make up the "total fat" listing on the label. These fats are outlined on the label as saturated fat, trans fat, polyunsaturated fat, and monounsaturated fat. The goal is to choose foods higher in unsaturated fat (monounsaturated fat, polyunsaturated fat), lower in saturated fat, and no (that's zero) trans fat. Although recent studies have deemed saturated fats as less harmful than previously believed, that doesn't necessarily make them beneficial. Until all the cards are laid out on the table, it's best to get your fat facts through the following descriptions of the three types of fats:

Unsaturated fat: Unsaturated fats are listed under total fat. These are fats that are liquid at room temperature. Foods high in unsaturated fat are vegetable oils, nuts, and fish. Unsaturated fats, like olive and canola oils, are often called "good fats" because they may not raise cholesterol levels as trans fats do.

Saturated fat: The amount of saturated fat appears beneath the total fat on the Nutrition Facts Panel. Saturated fat usually comes from animal products like butter, cheese, whole milk, ice cream, and meats. Saturated fat should account for less than 7-10 percent of your total calories for the day, which equates to 140 to 200 calories in a 2,000 calorie diet. Saturated fats and trans fats are often called "bad fats" because they could raise cholesterol and increase a person's risk for developing heart disease. Both saturated and trans fats are solid at room temperature.

Fast Fact

Even if a food product claims to have "0 grams trans fat" on the front of a package, be sure to flip to the ingredient list on the label to make sure there are no "partially hydrogenated fats" listed. Under the current [2016] guidelines, companies may claim that a product contains zero grams trans fat if it contains less than 0.5 grams per serving. Consistently choosing foods with even a minute amount of trans fat can add up to a significant trans fat intake if portion control isn't practiced.

Trans fat: Since 2006, food manufacturers also have been required to list trans fats separately on the label. Although trans fats are found naturally in some foods, like meats, butter, and whole milk, most trans fatty acids in the diet come from artificial partially hydrogenated fats that are manmade, such as shortenings and stick margarine. The hydrogenation process makes fats more stable, thereby extending their shelf life, but eating trans fats will not help extend your life. Quite the contrary: Trans fats raise harmful LDL ("bad") cholesterol levels and deplete protective HDL ("good") cholesterol levels. The body is unable to burn or use trans fats, causing them to build up and clog arteries that lead to the heart and brain.

Trans fats are even more dangerous than saturated fat because not only do they raise the type of cholesterol in the body that is considered to be "bad" (known as LDL cholesterol), but they reduce the "good" cholesterol (known as HDL cholesterol). This is why your trans fat intake should be zero.

Be on the lookout for all types of trans fats. In 2013, the FDA determined artificial partially hydrogenated oils [trans fats] are no longer "generally recognized as safe" [GRAS]. After a twoyear review period, the FDA finalized its determination about the negative health outcomes of artificial trans fat consumption and required manufacturers to eliminate trans fats from processed foods. By 2018, artificial trans fats will no longer be allowed in processed foods, such as cookies, crackers, coffee creamers, and more. As such, manufacturers have increased their use of saturated fats such as palm, palm kernel, and coconut oil in packaged foods.

When reading the Nutrition Facts Panel on your food label, the number you should look for next to trans fat is zero, but don't stop there…be sure to check the Ingredient List and avoid any hydrogenated fats.

Fast Fact

Your goal should not be to avoid fat, but to instead be sure that most of the fat in your diet comes from foods rich in unsaturated fat (e.g., monounsaturated fat, polyunsaturated fat), and limited in saturated fat. Trans fats (partially hydrogenated fats) should be ditched.

Cholesterol

This word became more popular than disco in the 70s. Everyone knew they should avoid it, but they didn't know what it was or where it was hidden in the foods they were eating. What you also may not know is that you can't live without it.

Cholesterol is a wax-like substance used by the body for many vital functions, including producing vitamin D and some hormones, and for building many other important substances. If your blood cholesterol levels are too high, however, your risk of heart disease or stroke increases.

Most of the cholesterol you need is manufactured by your liver. However, dietary sources such as meat and poultry, eggs, and whole-milk dairy products were believed to significantly contribute to cholesterol levels and the other laboratory values your doctor screens for when he or she checks your lipid profile through blood tests. A high blood cholesterol level can lead to a buildup of plaque in your arteries, called *atherosclerosis*, which can increase your risk of heart attack and stroke.

Although some people require medication to help lower cholesterol levels, it does not need to be your first line of defense. The 2015 *Dietary Guidelines for Americans* suggest reducing your saturated fat intake to less than 10 percent of total caloric intake and the American Heart Association suggests limiting saturated fat intake even further to less than 7% of total caloric intake to significantly lower blood cholesterol levels even more than reducing your dietary cholesterol intake. In fact, the 2015-2020 *Dietary Guidelines for Americans* no longer pinpoint an exact quantity of dietary cholesterol to limit in your diet as previous editions did.

Dietary cholesterol is only found in animal foods. On your food label, cholesterol is listed under the fat information and is measured in milligrams. Treat animal protein as a side dish and limit lean meat, fish, and poultry to no more than 6 ounces per day (a 3-ounce portion is about the size of a deck of playing cards), and you may want to try to avoid cholesterol-laden organ meats, such as liver, brains, and kidneys. Choosing plant proteins, like beans and nuts may not only not contribute cholesterol to your diet, but they may actually lower such levels.

Better oil choices for those watching their cholesterol are canola, sunflower, safflower, corn, soybean, olive, and peanut oils. You should also choose complex, whole-grain carbohydrates (certain fibers contained within oats and beans can lower your blood cholesterol levels), fish, and, of course, lots of fruits and vegetables.

Sodium

Sodium, a component of salt, is listed on the Nutrition Facts Panel in milligrams. Sodium helps with the transmission of electrical signals through nerves, and small amounts of sodium are necessary for keeping proper body fluid balance. Most Americans consume far too much sodium. That's no surprise when even cooking shows on TV highlight chefs dipping their hands into the salt dish and generously sprinkling salt into their creations, almost like the way farmers feed their chickens on the farm!

An excessive sodium intake can contribute to hypertension (high blood pressure) and stroke, and has also been linked to osteoporosis, kidney damage, and stomach cancer. It's no wonder why salt is becoming the new trans fat, earning it the title of "the silent killer."

Although almost all foods naturally contain small amounts of sodium, highly processed foods can be loaded with sodium. In an effort to control high blood pressure and reduce the risks of heart disease, it is recommended that we limit the amount of sodium we consume to an upper limit of 2,300 mg per day. (This value is for an average, healthy person—not necessarily the amount suggested for someone with hypertension, where the recommended upper limit of intake is 1,500 mg per day.) Although that may sound like a generous number, according to a national study, the average daily intake of sodium is almost double that amount. One of the culprits is the addition of extra salt to add some flavor to low-fat and low-sugar foods in an attempt to tantalize taste buds without the calories. Salt can lurk in seemingly innocent foods like breads, cereals, and crackers, as well as more obvious products like salted nuts, soups, olives, and convenience foods. As a frame of reference, an average pickle contains about 1,900 mg of sodium, a teaspoon of salt has 2,325 mg, and an average cup of soup can have 800 to 1,000 mg of sodium.

Here's where label reading is critical. Checking the sodium content of the foods you eat and keeping a mental tally of how quickly those numbers add up is important, but don't stop there; it's also important to pay attention to the serving size. As I mentioned before, if you eat more than the amount that's listed as a serving, you need to double or triple the milligrams of sodium consumed. I've seen cans of soup with labels that read "sodium—900 mg," but it may also list the number of servings per can as 2. That means that this one little can of soup is giving you more than two-thirds of the average sodium requirement for the entire day.

If you notice that the sodium content listed within the Nutrition Facts Panel of a product is high, and you don't see the word "salt" in the ingredient list, words like baking powder (480 mg sodium per teaspoon), baking soda (1,200 mg sodium per teaspoon), or any compound with sodium in its name, such as monosodium glutamate, could be the offender. Look for labels that state that the item is:

- Sodium-free (less than 5 mg sodium per serving),
- Very-low-sodium (35 mg or less per serving), or
- Low-sodium (140 mg or less per serving)

Even if a product is labeled "reduced sodium," it doesn't necessarily mean that it will be low enough in salt to meet your particular requirements. Just so you know, a food wearing the label "reduced sodium" means that it contains 25% less sodium than the original...but not that it is lowsodium! Aside from checking labels, you may need to consult with your physician or registered dietitian nutritionist to help coordinate your dietary and medical needs.

Fast Fact

It is recommended that the average healthy person limit the amount of sodium consumed to an upper limit of 2,300 mg per day. Some experts feel that number should be reduced to 1,500 mg. One pickle could have 1,900 mg.

Total Carbohydrate

Carbohydrates, fondly referred to as "carbs," have gotten a bad name, though our love affair with high-protein, low-carb diets seems to be waning. Although people enjoyed eating steaks bigger than the size of their plates, after the initial honeymoon was over, even a dry cracker started to look good.

The carbohydrate section on your label tells you how many grams of carbohydrates are in each serving of the food you are eating and the percentage of the Daily Value this represents. This number includes starches, complex carbohydrates, dietary fiber, added sugar sweeteners, and nondigestible additives.

Starches are polysaccharides, made up of long chains of glucose (sugar) molecules that are broken down more slowly than simple sugars. These carbs are found in whole-grain bread, cereal, pasta, potatoes, beans, rice, and starchy vegetables like corn. Complex carbs are rich in vitamins, minerals, fiber, and healthful phytochemicals, which may reduce the risk of cardiovascular disease and cancer while also keeping us more satiated. Carbs are also an excellent source of energy and are an important part of your daily diet. If you need to lose weight, you may need to pay closer attention to your portion sizes of carbohydrate-type foods, but don't avoid them completely. When it comes to carbs and weight, you might need to take a closer look at the company they keep: the baked potato may not be as much of an issue as the butter and sour cream you pile on top of it.

The following types of carbohydrates add up to the total carb value.

Fiber

Roughage, bulk, bloat, intestinal cleansing . . . sound attractive? Not really. These are words that are often associated with fiber, and maybe that's why most Americans are not getting enough of the stuff. But fiber is more than just a gastrointestinal plunger. Eating fiber has been shown to reduce the incidence of diabetes, heart disease, stroke, and cancer. Most high-fiber foods are also low in calories, and since eating more fiber can help you feel fuller for a longer period of time, it may also reduce the risk of obesity.

Recent studies have also shown that the right fibers provide fuel for the good bacteria that lives inside of us which could have a positive impact on everything from your immune system to the prevention of chronic diseases.

Americans are taking in about half the amount of fiber they need each day. The quantity of fiber you need depends upon your age and gender. The Institute of Medicine recommends an Adequate Intake (AI) of 38 grams a day for men up to age fifty, and 25 grams a day for women of that same age group. Although those numbers decrease to 30 grams for men and 21 grams for women from fifty-one-plus years of age, the fact is that our digestive tracts become more sluggish as we age, activity levels decrease, and the ability to detect when we're thirsty also diminishes. In other words, although the numerical requirement of fiber decreases with age, the *importance* of fiber increases with age, making it an essential dietary component later in life.

Most people don't realize how many ways fiber contributes to our health. Fiber prevents constipation, hemorrhoids, and diverticulosis, may reduce the incidence of colon and breast cancers, fuel gut bacteria, and may lower LDL (bad) cholesterol and stabilize blood sugar levels, thereby decreasing the risk of heart disease and diabetes. The government has permitted a health claim linked to fiber because of its role in reducing blood lipids (fats).

Fast Fact

Don't forget to get your daily fix of fiber! The FDA updated the daily value recommended for fiber to 28 grams per day, based on a 2,000 calorie per day diet. Most of us don't even come close to that amount!

You'll find fiber listed in grams on the label in the Nutrition Facts Panel as **Total Fiber**, which is defined as **dietary fiber** plus **functional fiber**. Here is a description of the two:

Dietary fiber is the fiber that's naturally present in plant-based foods. This form is the indigestible portion that moves food through the digestive system, absorbing water and promoting easier bowel movements. Dietary fiber consists of dextrins, inulin, lignin, waxes, chitins, pectins, gums, cellulose, beta-glucans, oligosaccharides, and some resistant starch. There are two types of dietary fiber, **soluble** and **insoluble**. These types differ based upon how they interact with water. Both types of fiber are present in all plant foods, with varying degrees of each according to a plant's characteristics.

Insoluble fiber is a natural laxative that attracts water and helps to increase bulk, soften stool, and shorten the time it takes for foods to move through the intestinal tract, known as transit time. Sources of insoluble fiber are foods made with whole wheat, bran, nuts, seeds, and the skin of some fruits and vegetables.

Soluble fibers offer significant health benefits, including supporting the immune system and normalizing blood sugar and cholesterol levels. These fibers dissolve in water to form a

Insoluble Fibers	Soluble Fibers
Whole wheat	Oats
Bran Nuts	Beans
Seeds	Legumes
Skin of fruits and vegetables	Bananas
Popcorn	Flesh of apples, pears, citrus fruits
Cabbage, lettuce	Barley
	Psyllium seeds

gel-like substance. Sources of soluble fiber are oats, legumes (beans, peas, and soybeans), apples, bananas, berries, citrus fruits, barley, some vegetables, pectin, and psyllium seeds.

Functional fiber includes nondigestible parts of plants (such as resistant starch, pectins, and gums), chitins, chitosans, or commercially produced fiber (such as polydextrose). Functional fiber refers to carbohydrates that have been extracted from plants. Like dietary fiber, functional fiber also slows the transit of food through the GI tract and helps us to feel fuller longer. This type of fiber is often added to products that do not naturally contain much fiber (like yogurt) to boost the products' health benefits.

A food containing 5 grams or more fiber per serving is considered to be "high" in fiber. A "good" source is 2.5 to 4.9 grams, and the addition of 2.5 grams of fiber or more added to a product allows it to claim that it has "more" or "added" fiber above what the original food contained. (So if 2.5 grams of fiber were added to a brand called Grandma's Yogurt, then that product could claim that it had *more* fiber than similar products without added fiber.)

Sugar: The Master of Disguise

If sugar were a movie star, it would be typecast as the villain.

We've known for years that we eat too much sugar and that this ingredient is a major player in the obesity story. But sugar does not act alone: It's often accompanied (in products) by fat and it rarely travels with many valuable nutrients. But sugar is only part of the problem when it comes to our obesity crisis and health woes. We need to cut down on sugar, but sugar, often demonized, is not the only culprit in poorly planned diets.

Sugars are found in most foods. Fruits contain simple sugars but also contain fiber, water, and vitamins, and an array of antioxidants which makes fruit a healthier choice.

Nutrition Facts

Serving Size 1 cup (236ml)
Servings Per Container 1

Amount Per Serving

Calories 80   Calories from Fat 0

	% Daily Value*
Total Fat 0g	0%
Saturated Fat 0g	0%
Trans Fat 0g	
Cholesterol Less than 5mg	0%
Sodium 120mg	5%
Total Carbohydrate 11g	4%
Dietary Fiber 0g	0%
Sugars 11g	
Protein 9g	17%

Vitamin A 10%   •   Vitamin C 4%
Calcium 30% • Iron 0% • Vitamin D 25%

*Percent Daily Values are based on a 2,000 calorie diet. Your daily values may be higher or lower depending on your calorie needs.

So, as an example, if you look at a label for skim milk, it will show you that 1 cup contains 11-12 grams of sugar. This sugar comes from lactose, a naturally occurring sugar. Although this may seem like a big number, if you check farther down the panel, you'll see that milk also contains protein, calcium, vitamin D and a host of other nutrients of value.

Figure 3. Nutrition Facts Panel for Skim Milk

The updated Nutrition Facts label will help you distinguish *added* sugars from *naturally occurring* sugars in foods, such as fruit and milk.

Added Sugars include the sugar that manufactures add to a product to enhance sweetness. Snack foods, candy, and soda often have excessive amounts of added sugars without offering any nutritional benefits, frequently referred to as consuming "empty calories." Although carbohydrates have just 4 calories per gram, the high sugar content in soft drinks and snack foods could skyrocket if you're not paying attention. The new Nutrition Facts Panel will now clearly state the grams and %DV of added sugars in a food product. For example, under "Total Sugars – 39g," a can of soda will also state "Includes 39g Added Sugars -- 13%." Labels for these sugared beverages could also be deceiving, so check the Nutrition Facts Panel to see how many *servings* are in the bottle or can before you pour. As a frame of reference, a teaspoon (or average packet) of sugar contains 4 grams of sugar, therefore an average can of soda can add a whopping 10 teaspoons of sugar to your diet.

In general, the closer the number of grams of "sugar" is to the "total carbohydrates" in each serving, the less nutritious it is. Here's an example: Let's say you're in the supermarket trying to decide between two cookies. One has 20 grams of total carbohydrate and 3 grams of sugar, and the other has 20 grams of carbohydrate and 12 grams of sugar. If you deduct the grams of sugar from the grams of total carbohydrate in both examples, the number that's left is the amount of healthier carbohydrates. In this case, the first cookie would produce a number of 17 (20 minus 3), while the other cookie would give a number of 8 (20 minus 12), so the first cookie is the better choice. There are exceptions to this rule, including milk, some yogurts, and "100 percent juice" because they contain natural sugars, but it is a good general guideline to keep in mind.

With the latest trend of going back to "natural" foods, without artificial colors and sweeteners, sugar may be back on consumers' shopping lists since yes, sugar is "natural," (a popular term you can't necessarily trust).

Reading the Nutrition Facts Panel and ingredient listing carefully is the only way that you'll be able to prevent being fooled by a manufacturer's code name for sugar (see the following list). Using these synonyms for sugar make the product seem more glamorous and healthier than if they used plain table sugar, but all of these versions listed below are recognized and metabolized by the body in a similar fashion to traditional sugar.

The Nutrition Facts Panel will also help you identify what type of sugar is actually in the product. A quick way to identify a sugar is to look for the words "syrup" or "sweetener," or words ending in the letters "ose." Whatever the name, look at the ingredient list and try to avoid or limit products that list sugar or its close relatives in the first three ingredients.

Other Ways to Spell "Sugar"

- Corn sweetener
- Corn syrup or corn syrup solids
- Dehydrated cane juice
- Dextrin
- Dextrose
- Fructose

- Fruit juice concentrate
- Glucose
- High-fructose corn syrup
- Honey
- Invert sugar
- Lactose
- Maltodextrin
- Maltose
- Malt syrup
- Maple syrup
- Molasses
- Raw sugar
- Rice syrup
- Saccharose
- Sorghum or sorghum syrup
- Sucrose
- Syrup
- Treacle
- Turbinado sugar
- Xylose

High-Fructose Corn Syrup (HFCS): HFCS is a sweetener made from corn. It supplies the same 4 calories per gram as table sugar and is used worldwide in hundreds of products, including soft drinks and processed foods. Just check your ingredient list and you'll probably find it listed on baked goods, fruit drinks, salad dressings, candies, gums, and syrups.

While this often-talked-about ingredient is far from being healthy, it is not the only culprit. It's not that different from table sugar. Sugar is composed of two simpler sugars (fructose and glucose), containing equal amounts (50 percent) of each. HFCS, on the other hand, contains 55 percent fructose and 45 percent glucose. Some people do, however, believe there are concerns regarding HFCS, including claims that its use is addictive and increases your chances of getting diabetes and of becoming obese. At this time, more research needs to be done before we know anything conclusive.

The bottom line is that HFCS and sugar both supply empty calories, void of any valuable nutrients, and products containing these ingredients should be limited or swapped out for healthier options.

Fast Fact

Although high-fructose corn syrup is far from healthy, it is not the only culprit. Sugar provides about the same amount of calories and appears in similar types of foods. You can probably assume that if the sugar content of the food is high…the nutrient value is low.

Artificial Sweeteners and Sugar Substitutes

Like it or not, artificial sweeteners are here to stay. According to a recent study published in the *Journal of the Academy of Nutrition and Dietetics*, consumption of low-calorie, non-nutritive sweeteners are on the rise for both children and adults. The study reports that between 1999 and 2012 adult consumption of low-calorie sweeteners increased 54% and consumption among children escalated by an enormous 200%! Study participants reported using low calorie sweeteners once daily, but daily use increased with adult body weight. In fact, the American Heart Association and American Diabetes Association have both released statements warning about use of artificial sweeteners as a weight loss tool. Due to the fact that artificial sweeteners are much sweeter than table sugar research has shown that continued use of artificial sweeteners hyper-stimulates our brains desire for sweet foods, which can contribute to weight gain.

The FDA must regulate and approve the use of artificial sweeteners and sugar substitutes. The FDA currently has five artificial sweeteners approved: acesulfame, aspartame, neotame, saccharin and sucralose. In spite of continued controversy as to whether the use of these products poses health risks, customers remain loyal to their colorful little packets. To make matters even more confusing, manufacturers are now mixing different sweeteners together, and even mixing some with sugar to keep the calories low but provide a smoother taste.

Here are the contenders:

- **Splenda:** Displayed in a yellow-colored packet, Splenda is recognizable name for the chemical sucralose, a derivative of the sugar molecule glucose. Sucralose is lower in calories than regular sugar, and it was approved by the FDA in 1998 for public use. Sucralose is up to six hundred times sweeter than regular sugar. One of the benefits of using this sweetener is that unlike other artificial sweeteners, you can bake with it without its composition changing, and it's sold in supermarkets in bulk packs to use in recipes.

- **NutraSweet/Equal:** This blue-colored packet often used as a sugar substitute in sodas is aspartame, and it is sold to the public under the names NutraSweet, Equal, and Spoonful. Aspartame is up to two hundred times sweeter than regular sugar and contains little to no calories. Aspartame was approved by the FDA in 1981, but its health risks are often in question, including complaints of severe headaches, methanol toxicity, and a possible cancer link. Those who suffer from PKU (phenylketonuria), a genetic disorder that is characterized by an inability of the body to utilize the essential amino acid, phenylalanine, must stay away from products containing aspartame. A warning label regarding this disease is by law required to be placed on all products containing aspartame. On sodas, this usually is on the back of the label, near the ingredient list. This product is not recommended for baking.

  The nutrition advocacy group Center for Science in the Public Interest has classified aspartame as a substance to be avoided.

- **Sweet'N Low:** The pink packet we've seen around for years contains the sweetener known as Sweet'N Low, made with saccharin. Saccharin is three hundred times sweeter than sugar. There has been much controversy surrounding Sweet'N Low and its possible cancer-causing effects. In fact, saccharin used to carry a warning label that linked it to cancer in rats; it was rescinded in 2000.

- **Ace-K:** Acesulfame-K is about two hundred times sweeter than sugar and is often added to soda in combination with other sweeteners (such as aspartame). The "K" refers to potassium.

- **Stevia/Truvia/PureVia:** Stevia is a sweetener extracted from the leaves of the stevia plant, called Rebaudioside A, Reb A, or Rebiana. It can be up to three hundred times sweeter than regular sugar and it contains no calories. Although stevia was first approved as a sweetener by the FDA in 2008, it has been used for hundreds of years in South America. Because it is derived from a plant, this product is being promoted as a "natural" sweetener, making it an increasingly popular choice.

- **Sugar Alcohols**: Sugar alcohols, such as xylitol, mannitol, and sorbitol, do not contain ethanol, as alcoholic beverages do. They appear naturally in foods like berries and plums, and you'll also find them in commercial products derived from glucose, sucrose, and starch, such as chewing gum, candy, frozen desserts, and more. Many consumers believe that these substances "don't count," but they can have an impact on blood glucose levels. Sugar alcohols are used as a sugar substitute, and contain about half to one-third fewer calories than regular sugar. They are metabolized more slowly than sugar, making them an attractive ingredient for people who have diabetes; however, some of the products they are in may still contain significant amounts of carbohydrates that need to be accounted for. Although these products are often used for weight loss purposes, over-consumption can lead to unwanted and unpleasant side effects, such as gas, bloating, and diarrhea. The declaration of sugar alcohols on food package labels is voluntary, so be sure to check the ingredient list – they usually end in –ol.

Fast Fact

Proceed with caution when consuming products that contain sugar alcohols, as they can cause diarrhea, flatulence, and gastrointestinal discomfort. You can spot sugar alcohols on the label, as most end in the
letters "ol," such as sorbitol and mannitol.

Protein

Protein is still the darling of the nutrients and most people just can't get enough of it. The protein group includes fish, poultry, meat, cheese, eggs, beans, nuts and seeds, and soy products. Over time, we have learned that our actual protein needs are far less than what most Americans consume on a daily basis. In fact, the 2015-2020 U.S. Dietary Guidelines for Americans stress that a healthy eating pattern includes only 5-½ ounces of protein foods per day (based on a 2,000 calorie per day meal plan). If you were to eat 1 tablespoon of peanut butter at breakfast, 2 hard boiled eggs in a salad at lunch, and 3 ounces of meat, poultry or fish at dinner, you would already exceed your required protein intake for the day.

It's not that the government suddenly decided to recommend slashing our "main dish" mentality; the guidelines were changed to reflect the portions of protein *actually needed*. It's difficult for some to think of protein as a side dish and not the centerpiece of the plate, and many people don't realize the wealth of protein available from nonmeat, plant-based sources like beans, nuts and seeds. The 2015-2020 Dietary Guidelines for Americans stress the inclusion of more plant foods in our overall diet, including protein sources, because these are often much lower in saturated fat and dietary cholesterol and may in fact, reduce cholesterol levels.

Protein is an essential nutrient for good health. Without sufficient protein, our bodies wouldn't be able to build lean, healthy muscle or perform important functions like protecting the immune system. Some protein sources are also high in fat and cholesterol, so finding the right balance and eating the right type of protein for a healthy body can be a challenge. Below are some guidelines to help you determine how much protein you should have in your daily diet.

Your Daily Protein Allowance

The Recommended Daily Allowance (RDA) of protein, according to U.S. government standards, is 0.8 gram per kilogram (2.2 pounds) of ideal body weight for adults, or about 0.4 gram of protein per pound. Between 10 to 15 percent of your total calories should come from protein. If, for example, you consume 2,000 calories per day, at least 200 calories (about 50 grams) should come from protein. There are some special circumstances where your protein needs may be greater, such as during pregnancy or for wound healing. Additionally, your protein requirements are also affected by your typical activity levels.

Below is a listing of the protein content of some common foods:

- 1 cup skim milk = 8 grams
- 1 egg = 6 grams
- ½ cup cottage cheese = 14 grams
- 1 ounce peanuts = 7 grams
- 6 ounces tofu = 12 grams
- 3 ounces sirloin steak = 26 grams

- ¼-pound hamburger patty = 28 grams
- 1 ounce cheese = 6 grams
- ½ cup beans = 6 grams

As you can see, you don't need to eat big portions to reach your recommendation for protein. Remember that moderation is always the key to healthy eating, even when you're talking about eating foods that are healthy for you. Many of us eat way beyond the amount of protein we need. Excessive protein consumption, particularly animal protein, can put your health at risk by placing a strain on your heart and increasing the risk of stroke, osteoporosis, and kidney stones. Highprotein fad diets can recommend up to four times the amount of protein you need and can cause you to lose more than weight: You can lose water, causing dehydration, as well as the valuable benefits of fiber and superfoods like fruits and vegetables. Moreover, the weight lost is often temporary, as these diets promote the avoidance of energy-rich carbohydrates to an unrealistic degree.

How many grams of protein are in an ounce of protein?

One of the most common yet confusing labeling questions I get asked is in relation to protein. Government recommendations are usually made in ounces (for example, the average woman needs 5 to 6 *ounces* of protein a day), but protein is listed on the label in grams. An important number to keep in mind is that **7 grams of protein = approximately 1 ounce of protein**. Therefore, if you were reading the label of your favorite veggie burger and it read: Protein 14 g, the burger would be equivalent to about 2 ounces of protein.

Percent Daily Values

Percent Daily Values (% DV) are listed in the right-hand column in percentages; they tell how much of a certain nutrient a person will get from eating *one serving* of that food. Ideally, the goal is to eat 100 percent of each of those nutrients each day by combining many different healthy foods together. For example, the DV for calcium is 1,300 mg. If one serving of a food contains

260 mg of calcium, the label would say that it contains a DV of 26 percent for calcium. In other words, one serving gives you 26 percent of the Daily Value for calcium.

Again, keep in mind that the Daily Values found on food labels are based upon consuming an average diet of 2,000 calories per day. For some nutrients, you may want to consume more or less than 100 percent of the DV, depending on your individual needs, such as pregnancy. The actual number of calories and nutrients required is going to vary according to your age, weight, gender, and level of physical activity. For more guidance on this, check with the USDA's My Plate at www.ChooseMyPlate.gov. This guide will help you assess your specific requirements. By checking the % DV, you can comparison shop and put two similar foods side by side to see how they measure up.

The Highs and Lows of Percent Daily Values

Percent Daily Value is most useful for determining whether a food is high or low in certain nutrients.

If a food has **5 percent or less** of the Daily Value of a nutrient, it is considered to be **low** in that nutrient.

If a food has **between 10 percent and 19 percent** of the Daily Value of a nutrient, it is considered to be a **good** source of that nutrient.

If the food has **more than 20 percent** of the Daily Value of a nutrient, it is considered **high** in that nutrient.

Remember that the % DV refers to a whole day, not to a single meal or snack.

Fast Fact

Keep in mind that the % Daily Values found on food labels are based upon consuming an average diet of 2,000 calories per day. Depending on your individual needs, you may want to consume more or less than 100 percent. For someone wanting to lose weight, 2000 calories per day could be too high, whereas if you're an athlete, the same amount of calories might fulfil only half of your needs. You can get the lowdown on what you need by logging on to www.ChooseMyPlate.gov.

The Ingredient List: "If I can't pronounce it . . . should I eat it?"

As a lawyer, my husband always talks about the importance of reading the "fine print." In my profession, the ultimate example of the fine print is the list of ingredients on a food label.

Ingredient declaration is required on all foods that have more than one ingredient.

Both FDA and U.S. Department of Agriculture (USDA) regulations require that food labels list each ingredient in descending order of weight. This simply means that the ingredient that weighs the most is listed first, and the ingredient that weighs the least is listed last. Ingredients are also supposed to be listed by their common, specific names.

For some people, the ingredient list is the most important part of the food label, especially for people who have food allergies or must avoid certain foods. Just by looking at a list, you might not know that caseinate, whey solids, and lactalbumin are all derived from cow's milk, or that hydrolyzed vegetable protein comes from wheat, peanuts, soybeans or other legumes.

The ingredient directory can be used as a guide to help you choose foods that are more nutritious (like whole grains), and it can also alert you to proceed with caution regarding ingredients that may be unhealthy or harmful (like partially hydrogenated fats). Thanks to the passage of the Food Allergen Labeling and Consumer Protection Act of 2004 (FALCPA),

33

consumers are better informed and feel more secure about the potential hidden dangers that could be lurking within the foods they purchase. Certain ingredients can be life-threatening to individuals with severe food allergies, while others may have food sensitivities to specific items that can result in uncomfortable symptoms. Precise ingredient information is also essential for those who need to keep a close eye on particular ingredients for religious or cultural reasons, or people who are vegetarians.

Whatever the case, consumers have a right to know that they will be able to make safe food choices without fear and uncertainty. The label must also list the FDA-certified color additives by name.

Food Additives

Food additives are any substances added to food used in its production, processing, treatment, packaging, transportation, or storage. All food additives are carefully regulated by federal authorities and various international organizations to ensure that foods are safe to eat and are accurately labeled. Many of these substances are not very complex and are not difficult to pronounce, like vanilla and baking soda, while others look like words you'd only see in the final round of a spelling bee.

Food additives and preservatives are often feared and shunned, but as you can see from the examples I just mentioned, many of these ingredients are not harmful and may in fact have protective qualities. Additives have been used throughout the ages, dating back to the use of salt to preserve meat and fish. Herbs and spices were used as flavoring agents, and natural colors from fruits and vegetables were relied on instead of the commercial products we use today.

Scores of new food and color additive petitions are submitted to the FDA each year. If approved, the FDA then issues regulations including the types of foods in which an additive can be used, the maximum amounts to be used, and how they must be identified on food labels. Authorization is also required by the USDA for use in meat and poultry products. Regulations known as Good Manufacturing Practices (GMP) limit the amount of food and color additives used, and as science changes, all additives are subject to ongoing safety reviews. The Delaney Clause, a provision of the Food Additives Amendment and the Color Additive Amendment, prohibits the approval of an additive if it is found to cause cancer in humans or animals. The two groups of substances that are exempt from the Food Additives Amendment are substances sanctioned by the FDA or USDA prior to 1958 and substances generally recognized as safe (GRAS). The GRAS list includes hundreds of additives that were exempt from the regulatory process, such as salt, sugar, monosodium glutamate (MSG), and spices, as scientific evidence deemed their use in food as being safe. Additives not considered as GRAS or prior approved must be approved before a product can go to market.

The consumer advocate group Center for Science in the Public Interest (CSPI) has been watching our backs for years, and even they agree that most additives are safe and that some even increase the nutritional value of the food. As a general rule, though, they believe we should "avoid sodium nitrite, saccharin, caffeine, olestra, acesulfame K, and artificial coloring." As far as they are concerned, "Not only are they among the most questionable additives, but they are used primarily in foods of low nutritional value." They encourage us to pay particular attention to "the two most familiar additives: sugar and salt," as "they may pose the greatest risk because we consume so much of them." For a comprehensive look at CSPI's list of food additives, refer CSPI's Chemical Cuisine in the Appendix.

The bottom line is that although there are over 3,000 different food additives that are approved by the FDA as being safe for human consumption, that doesn't mean that certain additives that are considered to be safe today won't wind up being chemicals that are <u>banned tomorrow</u>.

This Additive Will Really "Bug" You

The bursting red and yellow colors within your lemonade or ice cream may have come from an unlikely source: a bug. It comes in the form of the dried cochineal bug, labeled on your food as "artificial colors" or "color added." Thanks to the Center for Science in the Public Interest's campaign, the FDA imposed a rule that any food or cosmetic containing this bug (also known as carmine) needs to be labeled as such. Several dozen reports of adverse reactions to this critter spurred the change in ruling. Aside from being essential to those who have food allergies, labeling of insects in foods is particularly important to certain groups, including vegetarians, Jews, and Muslims.

Chapter 4

What Else Is On Your Label

Food Safety Issues

Without even having to think of a pickup line, every product in the supermarket gets a date. In fact, some items get multiple dates. These dates help consumers choose the freshest and safest foods available.

You might be shocked to hear that there is no uniform or universally accepted system used for food dating in the United States. Dating of certain foods is only required by a little more than half of our states, and there are actually areas of the United States where much of the food supply has some sort of open date and/or food isn't dated at all. Dates are not required by law—it is voluntary. The FDA regulates packaged foods and drugs, and only for infant formula does it require a use-by, or expiration, date. Infant formula is held to a high standard and each nutrient represented on the label must be at its peak nutrient value when sold. The USDA regulates fresh produce and meats.

Many of the dates used are not an indicator of safety but rather of quality.

Let's explore what you should look for in a date:

A **pack** date is the date the food was manufactured, processed, and packaged. This type of date is used for foods that have a longer shelf life, like canned or frozen goods. Frozen foods are best if used within a couple of months of this date. Canned goods can remain unopened for up to a year after this date. The date can be written as a month/day/year or referred to with a three-digit number starting from January 1 as 001, and ending with December 31 as 365.

The **pull-by** or **sell-by** dates are printed on dairy and meat products; this is the last date the product should be sold. It defines how fresh the product is. If stored properly, that date can be extended by a few days and the food may still be safe to consume, but the store should not be displaying the product past this date. If that date has passed, you should not buy the product.

Best-if-used-by (or before) dates are recommended to represent the products' best quality; after this date, the food may lose some of its freshness and nutritional value, but this is not a purchase or safety date. Eating the product after the date won't hurt you, but there might be some loss of flavor and quality. Cans exhibit a best-if-used-by date that connotes the date of peak quality. High-acid canned foods such as tomatoes, grapefruit, and pineapple can last twelve to eighteen months on the shelf. Foods of lower acidity, such as canned meat, poultry, fish, and vegetables, can last for two to five years if the can has been stored in a cool, dry, and clean place.

Expiration or **use-by** dates refer to the last date the food should be eaten or used. The date has been determined by the manufacturer of the product. Egg cartons are not required by federal law to use either a sell-by or expiration date, but they are required by some individual states. Egg cartons must display the "pack date," which defines when the eggs were washed, graded, and packaged. Purchase eggs before the sell-by or expiration date, and place them in their carton in the coldest part of your fridge, not on the door. They are their freshest if used three to five weeks from the date purchased. If the sell-by date expires over that time period, the eggs are still safe to use. Dating of baby food is for quality as well as for nutrient retention. Do not buy or use baby formula or baby food after its use-by date.

Open dating is found primarily on perishable foods such as meat, poultry, eggs, and dairy products. Open dates refer to the actual calendar dates, which are more easily interpreted by the average consumer, as opposed to the coded dating (see below) that was used in the past.

Closed, or **coded** dates are used by the manufacturer to identify and locate products; this is particularly helpful in the event of a recall. This type of dating might appear on shelf-stable products such as cans and boxes of food.

Bottom line: "When in doubt, throw it out." Every dietitian believes in the power behind this line. Don't eat anything that looks, smells, or tastes faulty.

The USDA, FDA, CDC, and others have created an online food safety headquarters for your convenience. Check out https://www.foodsafety.gov/ for a wealth of information regarding food safety and storage.

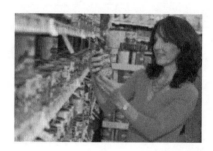

Glycemic Index

The **glycemic index**, or GI, is a measure of the effects of carbohydrates on blood glucose levels. Carbohydrates that break down quickly during digestion, releasing glucose rapidly into the bloodstream, have a high GI; carbohydrates that break down slowly, releasing glucose gradually into the bloodstream, have a low GI. This concept was developed by Dr. David J. Jenkins and colleagues in 1980 to 1981 at the University of Toronto in their research to find out which foods were best for people with diabetes.

For most people, foods with a low GI have significant health benefits. But that doesn't mean that this system is flawless. There are some relatively unhealthy foods that get a GI thumbs up, like premium ice cream, in part because of its high fat content because fat slows up the rate at which blood sugar is absorbed. The glycemic index of a food does not paint the whole nutrition picture: It does not give you any indication as to the amount of saturated or trans fat, the quality of the protein, or levels of vital nutrients within each food. Conversely, some foods, like carrots, for example, are loaded with positive nutrients, yet they don't score very well using this index because they are composed mostly of carbohydrates. But even if they don't rate as well, they shouldn't necessarily be cut out of your diet.

Moreover, the index ranks foods individually, so it does not give you the value of a food in the context of a whole meal. In other words, a teaspoon of jam might have a high glycemic index, but if a teaspoon of jam were put on a slice of whole-grain toast that was accompanied by a cheese omelet (rich in protein and fat), the index of the jam would be softened, and therefore it wouldn't have the same effect on blood sugar because foods high in protein and fat slow down the way carbohydrates are digested and absorbed. If you're trying to control your blood sugar and your weight, it might be best to count the amount and type (complex or refined) of carbohydrates you're eating.

Low GI Foods	High GI Foods
100% stone-ground whole wheat	White bread
Pasta	Short grain white rice
Beans and Lentils	Pumpkin
Sweet potatoes	Russet potatoes
Steel cut oats	Corn flakes, puffed rice cereal

Country of Origin Labeling (COOL)

Have you ever actually checked out the country-of-origin stickers on the foods you buy? When you start noticing these labels, you'll feel like you're in the United Nations instead of a grocery store. In 2009 and 2013, Congress passed laws requiring that labels on most fresh meats and some fruits, vegetables, as well as other foods must list where the food originated. In the case of meats, some labels will state where the animal was born, raised, and slaughtered. In 2015, the USDA repealed some of the previous laws, no longer requiring COOL labels for muscle cuts of beef and pork and ground beef or pork. According to the USDA, this rule covers muscle cut and ground chicken, lamb, and goat; wild and farm-raised fish and shellfish; perishable agricultural commodities (specifically fresh and frozen fruits and vegetables); peanuts, pecans, macadamia nuts, honey and ginseng. As far as fish and shellfish go, the method of production (whether farm-raised or wild) has to be written on the label. If the ingredient is an item in a processed food, it would be excluded from mandatory COOL. (Processed means that the food has undergone a physical or chemical change via a method such as cooking, curing, or smoking, or that has been combined with other foods.)

This COOL labeling (love that acronym) allows you to see how many miles your food had to travel before it got to your hands. Yellow peppers from Canada, grapes from Chile, or bananas from Ecuador—you can eat across the globe without leaving home, but is this a good thing?

Although free trade allows us to consume a bounty of food from foreign countries, travel increases the carbon footprint for food, which is not friendly for our environment. When produce travels a far distance, it may some lose nutritional value as well as taste. Consumers have a right to know where their food is coming from, but believe it or not, there are labels that read, "Product of Mexico, United States, or Canada." How informative is that?

Non-GMO

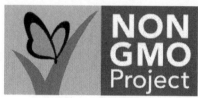

Figure 4. Non-GMO

GMOs (or genetically modified organisms) are organisms that have been created through the genesplicing techniques of biotechnology (also called genetic engineering, or GE). This science allows DNA from one species to be injected into another species in a laboratory, creating combinations of plant, animal, bacteria, and viral genes that do not occur in nature or through traditional crossbreeding methods. The majority of soybeans, corn, canola, sugar beets, and cotton grown in the United States are genetically modified for herbicide tolerance and insect resistance. Because of the prevalence of these crops as ingredients (particularly corn and soy), the FDA estimates that GMOs are currently in about 75-80% of processed foods. Until recently, there was no federal regulation requiring the presence of GMOs to be detailed on food labels, however, genetic modification is a "prohibited method" under the USDA's National Organic Program and until 2016, there was no federal government requirement for labeling of foods containing GM ingredients in nonorganic foods. In July 2016, a new law establishing a federal standard for transparency on food labels to state that they contain genetically modified organisms was created, but the precise rules, written by the Department of Agriculture, will not be set until 2018. This law is widely criticized, however, because it allows food companies to use QR codes or 1-800 numbers as a form of GMO labeling, which only makes it more difficult for consumers, requiring an extra step to get this information.

The use of GM foods has its potential advantages and disadvantages and the genetic modification of food is not new. This biotechnology helps crops thrive even during adverse conditions, such pest-resistant crops may lessen the need for any additional chemicals and pesticides, and foods produced may be more plentiful and cost effective. Some have argued that there may be greater costs, however, that GM foods bring that we don't know about, such as the effects of long-term use of these products. Other issues include the possible evolution of insects that are resistant to pesticides, the possible allergic reactions some people may develop from using GM foods, and the effect GM crops could have on the environment, possibly harming species that they may not have intended to effect.

But be on the lookout: Coming to a supermarket near you, many products will soon have a way for you to determine if GMOs are contained in that product, if they don't already wear a non-GMO verification seal.

Kosher Symbols

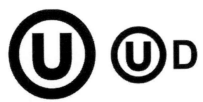

Figure 5. Kosher Certification Symbol from Orthodox Union (left) and Kosher-Dairy Certification Symbol from Orthodox Union (right)

Kosher symbols: The Hebrew word *kasheir*, or *kosher*, means "fit," or "proper." With regard to food, the above symbols indicate that a product is fit for consumption according to Jewish law. Kosher animals must have split hooves and chew their cud, like cows for example. Kosher fowl include chicken, turkey, and goose. Animals and fowl must be slaughtered by a specialist, called a shochet, and then soaked and salted. Nonkosher animals include pig, camel, and rabbit. All carnivorous (meat-eating) animals and fowl, the blood of these animals, and any derivatives or products thereof, are not considered to be kosher.

In the not-too-distant past, prepackaged kosher food, kosher restaurants, and kosher cookbooks were scarce. Today, kosher food has become a $12.5-billion-a-year business, strictly monitored by an intricate certification system. The largest system, called the Orthodox Union, places their OU symbol on kosher products, reflecting their supervision of both the ingredients and equipment used by food companies. Over 800,000 products are certified OU. Surprisingly, more than 70 percent of kosher-food consumers in the United States are not observant Jews. So why are these people purchasing kosher products?

According to a survey by Mintel, those who buy kosher do so because of food quality, general healthfulness and food safety. Kosher foods are believed to be "cleaner" and safer, with their food labels considered to be more strictly watched over owing to religious stipulations. This is particularly attractive to those with food allergies or sensitivities. As an example, if you have a seafood allergy, you can rest assured that crustaceans like lobster and shrimp will *never* be included in a kosher product. Non-kosher fish such as swordfish, catfish, eel, shark, and underwater mammals and reptiles are not permitted either. If you are lactose intolerant, you can be confident that foods that contain the word *parve* do not contain meat or dairy.

Parve foods include fish with fins (such as halibut and salmon) and all fruits, grains, and vegetables in their natural state. Not all kosher foods are parve, as many kosher foods contain meat or dairy. If the OU symbol is followed by a "D," it means that the product contains dairy and would not be lactose-free. If you are kosher, dairy products may not be eaten in combination with meat or fowl.

Fast Fact

Although kosher foods are believed to be "cleaner," because of their strictly regulated label system governed by religious rules, this does not mean that kosher foods are *healthier*. People who buy kosher foods have to carefully balance their diets and read labels just as closely as anyone else. If, however, you have food allergies or sensitivities such as lactose intolerance, kosher food labels can be trusted.

Zabihah Halal symbol

Halal is an Arabic word meaning lawful. Packages that display the halal symbol signify that the products conform with Islamic dietary law and are prepared and federally inspected accordingly. Similar to a kosher certification, a halal certification is provided by a qualified third party agency, however there is not one accepted symbol. Halal food is not necessarily kosher, nor is the opposite true. The symbol does however provide assurance that the contents of the food are not *forbidden*, known as *haram*. In order for processed foods to be considered halal, they must be free or pork and alcohol and must not have come in contact with such products. Meat and poultry must be slaughtered according to specific Islamic guidelines to be considered halal, and no food may touch or be contaminated in the storage or preparation process with meat that has not been properly slaughtered. Although fish is a part of the Muslim diet, certain shellfish, like prawns, may not be permitted by certain communities.

Chapter 5

Organic Food: Is It Worth It?

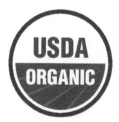

Figure 7. USDA Organic Symbol

Joni Mitchell was ahead of her time when she discouraged the use of pesticides in her song "Big Yellow Taxi" in 1970. Now, almost five decades later, we still have similar concerns, in addition to an increased consciousness of how our climate has changed.

A 2016 Gallop poll showed that 65 percent of Americans – the highest numbers in eight years -- believe that human activities contribute to climate change and that they worry a "great deal" or a "fair amount" about the impact climate change has on our environment. Nearly the same amount of Americans also believe that some change in lifestyle is necessary to combat climate change. According to the Food and Agriculture Organization of the United Nations, organic farming practices have "many advantages and considerable potential for mitigating and adopting to climate change."

With a rise in consumer awareness of the need to protect our environment along with an increased desire to protect our bodies through "cleaner" diets, organic food sales are skyrocketing around the globe. Across the country there are complete supermarkets that have dedicated their shelf space to healthy foods, and just about every mainstream store carries organic food, including their own private labels.

But do consumers even know what they are looking for? In a national survey conducted by the Shelton Group, when asked, "Which is the best product description to read on a label?" Americans chose "natural" over "organic" even though "natural" has never been officially defined by the Food and Drug Administration (FDA). The same cannot be said for the "organic" label, which must meet strict government standards to be certified as such.

The Definition of "Organic"

The International Federation of Organic Agriculture Movements (IFOAM) World Board has proposed a definition of organic agriculture as follows: organic foods have been produced without the use of synthetic pesticides, herbicides, fungicides, or synthetic fertilizers, and cannot be genetically modified or radiated. Organic poultry, dairy, meat, and eggs are produced without the use of growth hormones or antibiotics, and are humanely raised and slaughtered.

The Organic Foods Production Act and the National Organic Program (NOP) ensure that organic foods purchased in the United States are produced, processed, and certified to consistent national organic standards. On food labels, products that use the term "organic" must meet the following guidelines.

- Products labeled as "**100 percent organic**" must contain only organically produced ingredients (excluding water and salt).
- Products labeled "**organic**" must consist of at least 95 percent organically produced ingredients (excluding water and salt).
- "**100 percent**" and "**95 percent**" organic products must use the seal pictured above.
- Processed products that contain at least 70 percent organic ingredients can use the phrase "**made with organic ingredients**" and list up to three of the organic ingredients or food groups on the principal display panel.
- Products with less than 70 percent organic ingredients may only list those ingredients that are organic on the information panel.

The big question is whether organic foods are healthier and worth paying the premium for. For some time, the research about whether organic foods are nutritionally superior than their conventionally grown counterparts was questionable. Within the last few years, however, more research demonstrates that there are some significant nutritional benefits of choosing certain organic products over others. However, just because a food is labeled "organic" doesn't mean it gets to wear an automatic neon sign, glowing with the words "healthiest option." There are organic foods that are wholesome and healthful, and there are organic foods loaded with fat, sodium, and sugar (organic chips, cookies and candy, for example). **When buying organic, don't cast aside all other principles of healthy eating.**

Fast Fact

Official definition of organic agriculture: Organic foods have been produced without the use of synthetic pesticides, herbicides, fungicides, or synthetic fertilizers, and cannot be genetically modified or radiated. Organic poultry, dairy, meat, and eggs are produced without the use of growth hormones or antibiotics, and are humanely raised and slaughtered. This definition does not, however, reflect the nutritional value of the food.

Is It Worth the Switch?

Pros:

- Although some organic foods provide more nutrition-related benefits than their conventional counterparts, all organic foods are made without potentially harmful pesticides, fertilizers, antibiotics, synthetic hormones, or genetic engineering. A decrease in pesticide residues can be especially beneficial for children and at-risk populations such as pregnant women.

- Organic dairy and meat contain up to 50 percent more beneficial omega 3 fatty acids than conventionally produced dairy and meat.

- Organic producers cannot feed parts of any other animal to their cattle or chickens. Bovine spongiform encephalopathy (BSE), commonly known as mad cow disease, is a fatal illness that affects the nervous system of adult cows. This disease could be transferred to other cows if the animal feed is made from the infected part of the animals. The use of animal brain and spinal cord material in feed given to cattle, sheep, and goats has been banned by the FDA since 1997, and an extension of this ban to chicken feed is being considered.

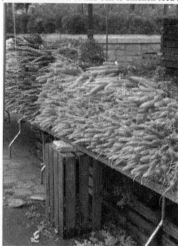

- Organically grown produce such as carrots, broccoli and blueberries contained substantially higher concentrations of antioxidants according to a 2014 meta analysis published in the *British Journal of Nutrition.*

- Locally grown organic produce in season can be comparable in cost to conventional produce. Additional benefits of local produce include increased support for local farmers, greater vitamin and mineral retention in foods (since your food doesn't have to travel far to get to your supermarket), and a pat on the back for the environment.

- Synthetic fertilizers and pesticides used in conventional farming account for almost 40 percent of the energy used in all of U.S. agriculture.
- Although taste is subjective, some people feel that organic food tastes better.

Cons:
- "Organic" doesn't necessarily mean that the food is grown locally—it may be grown in a foreign country and shipped to the United States, which results in a larger carbon footprint and smaller benefit to the environment, if any. Moreover, the organic label does not mean that such food is harvested from animals that were humanely treated or handled by workers that were receiving fair wages. It is meant to describe farming methods that are believed to be better for the land and producing healthier food.
- It also doesn't guarantee that the food was produced under ideal conditions for livestock or laborers.
- You'll probably have to put down more green to go green. Organic foods can cost up to 50 percent more than their nonorganic counterparts. The priority is to eat more fruits and vegetables—no matter which type you choose. Don't take a pass on this food category if the organic options are bursting your budget.
- Organic certification technically has nothing to do with food safety. The organic seal does not protect against salmonella, E. coli, or any other pathogens.

The bottom line is that you don't have to go home and empty every shelf in your cabinets and fridge to bring organic food into your diet. Start small, perhaps buying organic meat, poultry, and dairy. Organically grown meat and poultry are environmentally friendly, they are humanely raised, and they are fed organic grain. When it comes to fruits and vegetables, we have a hard enough time meeting our daily quota, so it's important to consume *any* produce.

The Environmental Working Group (EWG) devised a list of 12 fruits and vegetables – the "Dirty Dozen" -- that they consider to contain the most pesticides and are best to purchase organic [see below]. Some people feel that, when possible and affordable, it may be best to avoid the conventional "dirty dozen" and switch to organic for these twelve produce items. But not everyone agrees with the annual list released from the EWG, and many people, including health and nutrition professionals, feel that their lists will create fear and keep people away from consuming the essential fruits and vegetables that are already not getting enough of. Additionally, the EWG releases an annual "Clean Fifteen" list that details the 15 fruits and veggies that contain the *least* number of pesticides and are safest to buy from conventional farming methods.

In my opinion, the value of the rich nutrients within produce is something that should be trying to consume on a daily basis – organic or otherwise.

To save some money, try purchasing private label organic products instead of those that come from name brand manufacturers.

But most important, include lots of variety in your diet to limit your exposure to any one type of pesticide residue. Try to stick with produce that is subject to USDA regulations; pesticides used in other countries may not be allowed here. And moreover, look beyond the organic label—the number one priority to keep in mind is the product's total nutritional package, looking at saturated fat, trans fats, sodium, sugar, and calories, and consider how this particular food plays a role in your diet.

Green and Environmentally Friendly Food Packaging

A wholesome-looking, earth-friendly package surrounding a food does not necessarily mean that the food inside the package is wholesome or healthy. That would be like thinking that a car that looked good on the outside would work perfectly. Not true.

But as people all around the world become increasingly aware of the many environmental issues we face, the need to "go green" has become a new fashion statement worn everywhere, including in supermarkets. To hold our groceries, plastic bags are being replaced by biodegradable bags and reusable bags brought from home. Environmentally friendly food packaging alternatives are soaring. In fact, about 62 percent of shoppers claim that the green packaging of a product influences their decision in buying the product. But just as labels about food can be confusing and misleading, so can the public's interpretation of what "green" really means.

Although plastic has been a part of our lives for more than one hundred years, in some cases, its impact on the environment has been catastrophic. There are seven different types of plastic that you'll find in the supermarket, including those used for soft drinks, milk, meats, squeeze bottles, take-out meals, plates, and utensils. The most publicized and potentially dangerous plastic used is called *bisphenol A*, or BPA, so don't be surprised if you see labels on bottles indicating "this bottle is BPA-free."

You should be looking for:

- Environmentally friendly plastic. Food labels may make statements reflecting that suppliers are using "50% less plastic," and in many cases, consumers can actually feel the difference in the bottle; the plastic is much softer and tends to compress more easily. • Cornstarch and other agricultural commodities to replace petroleum-based plastic. Corn is now being used to make a compound known as polylactic acid, or PLA, which reportedly uses 65 percent less plastic than regular plastic containers, and it can decompose in a shorter time than conventional plastic. Although PLA still has its share of problems when it comes to being biodegradable (they require commercial composting facilities or other composts that must reach specific temperatures and humidity), experts agree that it is better for food packaging than petroleum-based plastics.
- Bottles that wear smaller labels, thereby using less paper (or even better, try the tap instead of bottled water).
- Paper products made from recycled paper and/or biodegradable packaging.

Just remember, you're not eating the package, so don't think that a new label and a new package on your bag of candy will make that same old product any healthier.

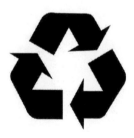

Figure 8. Chasing Arrows

The above "chasing arrows" symbol is the internationally recognized universal recycling symbol, composed of three chasing arrows that form an unending loop. There are many variations on this symbol, some accompanied by numbers. The lower the number, the easier it is to recycle the product, and other numbers reflect percentages (the portion of the item made up of recycled materials). These numbers appear on labels to help consumers paint a clearer picture about just how "green" their package is. Although this symbol is not a trademark, it is there to help us identify which products we can recycle.

Chapter 6

The Claim Game: Separating Fact from Fiction

Many product labels out there can be misleading, perhaps because we don't always know how to interpret what the labels are saying. Researchers repeatedly demonstrate that difficulties with math and reading significantly limit people's ability to adequately understand the information presented on food labels. Studies indicate that consumers have difficulty interpreting and using quantitative information on the Nutrition Facts Panel such as serving sizes and percent daily values, especially as these relate to daily intake recommendations. Quantitative errors when translating a food label can, of course, lead to both overestimation and underestimation of the amount of calories and nutrients consumed.

Grocery shopping should not be confusing or frustrating. Supermarkets, manufacturers, and consumers should be like the three legs on a stool, working in concert with each other to encourage a balanced diet and stable state of health. Food labels should represent the link between all groups, helping supermarkets showcase their goods, enabling manufacturers to inform shoppers about what's contained within their products, and educating consumers about how to make sensible food choices. Unfortunately, however, these parties are not always working in harmony.

On some days, I feel like I need a library card to take out foods from the store, since I spend so much time reading during my shopping experience. But what happens if you don't have the time to shop, like most multitasking consumers, or you don't get pleasure from being in the supermarket and you just want to make a quick, healthy purchase and exit? How can you make the best choice when you are bombarded with a multitude of food symbols of all different shapes, sizes, and . . . meaning? Many supermarkets now employ a registered dietitian nutritionist to help educate the public, but there's so much to learn that you may feel like you need a personal dietitian to walk you through the supermarket on every shopping trip! Plus, within the same store there may be other tags, signs, posters, and other educational systems that provide conflicting information. Sound confusing? Well, read on, and perhaps I can help walk you down the aisle.

Is It All in a Name?

To provide consumers with the products they are looking for, manufacturers often hook onto buzzwords that are frequently used in media stories, like "antioxidants," "natural," and "organic," and they use terms meant to attract shoppers like magnets, such as "no trans fat," "98% fat free," and "light," to name a few. Prior to the Nutrition Labeling Education Act [1990], the scrutiny of the meaning of these terms was left up to each individual consumer, each with varying interpretations; there was no universal standard definition. The FDA's ruling was meant to be very specific, consistent, and well-defined. This doesn't mean, however, that the information you'll see on packages is not confusing, ambiguous, or misleading. In the sections below, we'll first review the facts . . . and then we'll explore some fiction.

Labeling Claims

Once nutrient and health claims were allowed on food packages, manufacturers took the box and ran with it. According to the FDA, health claims apply to healthy subjects. The potential benefits of such claims are meant to encourage weight maintenance (and not necessarily promote weight loss), and should be based upon realistic portion sizes, which we already know is not necessarily the practice (but will hopefully change when the updated labels are released in 2018).

Although the following pages may seem a bit overwhelming, they're not meant to confuse you. Definitions need to be clear and unambiguous so that manufacturers don't look for loopholes and try to deceive unknowing shoppers. You don't have to memorize the following definitions; just use them as a source of reference when trying to figure out what the claim on your package really means. We will be taking a closer look at four different types of claims: **nutrient content claims, health claims, qualified health claims, and structure/function claims.**

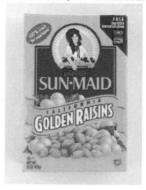

Nutrient Content Claims

If you're ever wandering down the aisles of the supermarket and see similar products, like bread for example, with "Low in Fat" displayed across the front of one package, "Low Sodium" stamped on another and "High Fiber" on a third, you're reading nutrient content claims. A nutrient content claim (NCC) describes the amount of nutrients (fat, cholesterol, fiber, etc.) within a food, without giving a specific number on the front of the package.

This claim cannot look as if it's surrounded by neon lights; a NCC can be no more than twice the size of the name of the food. In addition, a disclosure statement is required for nutrient content claims (e.g., low sodium, fat-free, sugar-free) if other nutrients within the food exceed certain thresholds (see the chart below). A disclosure statement alerts consumers to one or more nutrients in the food that may increase the risk of a disease or health-related condition that may be diet related. In other words, the disclosure statement identifies the nutrient that is present above the prescribed level (e.g., "See nutrition information for cholesterol content").

The disclosure statement must be on the label (immediately adjacent to the claim) when a claim is made and the food contains one or more of the following nutrients in excess of the levels listed below:

Total fat	13 grams
Saturated fat	4 grams
Cholesterol	60 mg
Sodium	480 mg

Meals and Main Dishes

Whether a main dish or meal-type product can make a nutrient content claim or health claim depends upon its contents. The product may not exceed the FDA's maximum nutrient levels for fat, saturated fat, cholesterol, or sodium as follows:

Meal-type products may not have more than:

Total fat	26 grams
Saturated fat	8 grams
Cholesterol	120 mg
Sodium	960 mg

Main dish products cannot have more than:

Total fat	19.5 grams
Saturated fat	6 grams
Cholesterol	90 mg
Sodium	720 mg

Any product represented as or considered to be consumed as breakfast, lunch, or dinner is subject to the special rules for "meal" products. Examples include frozen dinners or certain pizzas.

Claims that a meal or main dish is "free" of a nutrient, such as sodium or cholesterol, must meet the same requirements as those for individual foods.

"Low" claims can be made if the main dish or meal has:

- 120 calories or less per 100 grams,
- 140 mg sodium or less per 100 grams,
- 3 grams fat or less and no more than 30 percent of calories from fat per 100 grams
- 1 gram saturated fat or less and no more than 10 percent calories from saturated fat per 100 grams, *or*
- 20 mg cholesterol or less per 100 grams and no more than 2 grams of saturated fat per 100 grams.

Who You Gonna Call?

As a consumer, I called the FDA to find out what I should do in the event that I had a complaint about a particular product. In an interview with one of their consumer safety officers, I was able to find out the answers to some questions that I'd like to share with you.

Q: What should a consumer do if they find a product that carries a misleading label? A: If a consumer picks up a package carrying a label that they believe contains a claim that is not supported by the numbers on the Nutrition Facts Panel or the ingredient statement or any other label statement that they believe is wrong, the best thing to do is to contact the <u>Consumer Complaint Coordinator</u> (CCC) in their local FDA Office. Often people send complaints directly to FDA headquarters; in that case, we will assess the complaint and make a decision about whether there is enough information to evaluate, whether this is something that needs follow-up, and whether we need to send the complaint to our field office to investigate. When field investigators conduct routine inspections of food facilities, as well as checking for safety issues, they also look at product labels. Consumers can also contact the firm [food manufacturer] themselves because there may be a legitimate explanation for their label.

Q: What information does a consumer need to report if they are going to complain about a product or label?

A: Sometimes when consumers send in label complaints, they don't provide us with enough information to evaluate the complaint. For example, they may just mention the name of the product and tell us the problem. We encourage consumers that send in complaints about a food label to include the name of the food, the manufacturer's name, and if at all possible a copy of the food label in addition to the problem. (You can mail the actual label, take a picture of it, or scan it and e-mail it electronically.) This will help us expedite the review of the product label and determine what follow-up is appropriate.

Q: Do you receive many consumer complaints about products?

A: I don't know the exact numbers. We want to encourage consumers to continue to send in labels that they believe are incorrect. Some good sources of incorrect labels come from consumers.

Q: The FDA focuses a lot of its time and energy on food safety issues, and rightfully so. Do you think more attention is needed in the area of food labeling?

A: Inaccurate food labeling can also be a safety issue, for example, failure to declare an allergen. The <u>Office of Nutrition, Labeling and Dietary Supplements</u> has a division dedicated to food labeling issues. The office supports the development of a food labeling compliance program that sets FDA priorities for food labeling regulatory activities. This year a top priority for the FDA is food allergen labeling.

Definitions of Common Terms: Dealing with the Highs and Lows

Regulations spell out which terms may be used to describe the level of a nutrient in a food and how they can be used when employing claim terms such as "light," "reduced," "less," "fewer," "more," or "added." Here are the specifics of terms that are routinely displayed on foods we see every day. Alternative spelling of these descriptive terms and their synonyms is allowed—for example, "hi" and "lo"—as long as the alternatives are not misleading.

Free

This term means that a product contains no amount of, or only trivial or "physiologically inconsequential" amounts of, one or more of these components: fat, saturated fat, cholesterol, sodium, sugars, and calories.

Calorie-free: fewer than 5 calories per serving

Sugar-free and **fat-free**: less than 0.5 gram per serving

Synonyms for "free" include "without," "no," and "zero." Another name for fat-free milk is skim milk.

Food can only carry this "free" claim if it has been specially processed, altered, formulated, or reformulated so as to lower the amount of nutrient in the food, remove the nutrient from the food, or not include the nutrient in the food (e.g., "fat-free yogurt"). Foods that belong to the same food group (like vegetables) may make a statement identifying them, such as "carrots, a fat-free food." But a bag of carrots, for example, couldn't wear a label declaring that it is "fat-free," because carrots never have any fat in them to begin with.

"Fresh"

Although not mandated by the NLEA, the FDA has issued a regulation for the term "fresh," because of concern over the term's possible misuse on some food labels.

The regulation defines the term "fresh" when it is used to suggest that a food is **raw** or **unprocessed**. In this context, "fresh" can be used only on a food that is raw, has never been frozen or heated, and contains no preservatives, except:

- The addition of approved waxes or coatings,
- the post-harvest use of approved pesticides,
- the application of a mild chlorine wash or mild acid wash on produce, or • the treatment of raw foods with ionizing radiation

"Fresh frozen," "frozen fresh," and "freshly frozen" can be used for foods that are quickly frozen while still fresh. Blanching (before freezing to prevent nutrient breakdown) is allowed. The term "quickly frozen" is permitted as well (freezing via a system such as blast-freezing).

Good Source

Calling a food a "good source" means that one serving of that food contains between 10 and 19 percent of the Daily Value for a particular nutrient. So when it comes to fiber, for example, a serving of garbanzo beans (chickpeas) could be considered to be a good source since it contains 4 grams of fiber for ½ cup or 16% daily value.

Healthy

Some claims beg to be revisited. A "healthy" food, according to the definition established over twenty years ago, should be low in fat and saturated fat and contain limited amounts of cholesterol and sodium. So, would salmon, nuts, avocado and olive oil be unhealthy? This is a term that will surely be revisited in the near future, particularly since the importance of fat and fat-containing foods has been clearly established.

If it is a single-item food, like bread (as compared with a meal like a frozen dinner), it must provide at least 10 percent of one or more of vitamins A or C, iron, calcium, protein, or fiber. Exempt from this "10 percent" rule are certain raw, canned, and frozen fruits and vegetables and certain cereal-grain products. If it's a meal-type product, it must provide 10 percent of two or three of these vitamins or minerals or of protein or fiber, in addition to meeting the other criteria. The sodium content cannot exceed 360 mg per serving for individual foods and 480 mg per serving for meal-type products. There are many frozen dinners that contain colorful vegetables and lean protein as well as other "healthy" ingredients, but if, for example, they carry a sodium content of 1,000 mg, the product may not wear a "healthy" claim.

Of note, this also applies to related terms related terms "health," "healthful," "healthfully," "healthfulness," "healthier," "healthiest," "healthily" and "healthiness."

Fast Fact

Although your cooking spray doesn't appreciably add any fat during meal preparation, it cannot claim to be "fat-free," since it is essentially 100 percent fat. It does technically qualify for such a claim, but the label would then have to disclose that the product is 100 percent fat so as not to be misleading or confusing. That's why you'll see "for fat-free cooking" on the can instead of simply "fat-free."

High

This term can be used if the food contains 20 percent or more of the Daily Value for a particular nutrient in a serving. Orange juice, for example, is considered to be high in vitamin C, since one serving provides 120 percent of the day's Daily Value based upon a 2,000-calorie diet. In order to be considered "high fiber," a food must contain 5 grams of fiber or more per serving, so ½ cup of cooked navy beans (9.5 grams of fiber) is high in fiber.

Implied

Claims that wrongfully imply that a food contains or does not contain a meaningful level of a nutrient are prohibited. For example, a product claiming to be made with an ingredient known to be a source of fiber (such as "made with oat bran") is not allowed unless the product contains enough of that ingredient (oat bran) to meet the definition for "good source" of fiber. In addition, a claim that a product contains "no tropical oils" is allowed—but only on foods that are low in saturated fat because consumers have come to equate tropical oils with high saturated fat.

Lean and Extra-Lean

These terms can be used to describe the fat content of meat, poultry, seafood, and game meats.
> **Lean**: less than 10 grams fat, 4.5 grams or less saturated fat, and less than 95 mg cholesterol per serving and per 100 grams
> **Extra-lean**: less than 5 grams fat, less than 2 grams saturated fat, and less than 95 mg cholesterol per serving and per 100 grams

Less

This term means that a food, whether altered or not, contains 25 percent less of a nutrient or of calories than the reference food. For example, pretzels that have 25 percent less fat than potato chips, which are considered a similar food, could carry a "less" claim. "Fewer" is an acceptable synonym.

Light

This descriptor can mean two things:

First, a nutritionally altered product that contains one-third fewer calories or half the fat of the original food. An example of this would be "light" bread at 40 calories per slice, as compared with a similar slice of bread at 80 calories per slice.

Second, this term might mean that the sodium content of a low-calorie, low-fat food has been reduced by 50 percent. In addition, "light in sodium" may be used on food in which the sodium content has been reduced by at least 50 percent. "Light" soy sauce then would have to contain half the sodium of regular soy sauce. But if you're watching your sodium, be aware that even light soy sauce contains more than 1,000 mg of sodium per tablespoon. Be careful about what you're dipping your sushi into!

The term "light" still can be used to describe properties such as texture and color, as long as the label explains the intent—for example, "light brown sugar" and "light and fluffy." This term, however, is often taken too *lightly*. For example, "light" olive oil contains the same calories and fat as a thick, dark, rich, heavy olive oil—it just has a lighter-tasting flavor and a lighter color.

Low
Manufacturers can use the term "low" if the food can be eaten frequently without exceeding dietary guidelines for one or more of the following components:

Low-fat: 3 grams or less per serving
Low–saturated fat: 1 gram or less per serving
Low-sodium: 140 mg or less per serving
Very–low sodium: 35 mg or less per serving
Low-cholesterol: 20 mg or less and 2 grams or less of saturated fat per serving **Low-calorie**: 40 calories or less per serving

Synonyms for "low" include "little," "few," "low source of," and "contains a small amount of."

More
This term means that a serving of food, whether altered or not, contains a nutrient that is at least 10 percent of the Daily Value more than the regular version of the food. The 10 percent of Daily Value also applies to "fortified," "enriched," "added," "extra," and "plus" claims, but in those cases, the food must be altered.

Percent Fat-Free
A product bearing this claim must be a low-fat or a fat-free product. In addition, the claim must accurately reflect the amount of fat present in 100 grams (about 3 ounces) of the food.

Reduced
This term means that a nutritionally altered product contains at least 25 percent less of a nutrient or of calories than the regular version of the product. Pay attention here! A label may say that the food is reduced fat or reduced sodium, but **do not assume that this modification makes the product a low-fat or low-sodium product.** For example, if the regular version of a can of soup contains 1,200 mg of sodium per cup serving, and the "reduced" version contains 600 mg of sodium for the same quantity, then the reduced-sodium product would still be a high-sodium food. Moreover, a reduced claim can't be made on a product if its reference food already meets the requirement for a "low" claim, as listed above (for sodium, 140 mg or less per serving).

Manufacturers may use the terms "less," "fewer," or "more" in comparing products that have nothing to do with each other. They're supposed to be comparing "product categories," and not trying to match up two completely different classes of food. For example, it would be misleading to say, "broccoli has less fat than butter." These are not categories of food that would be considered to be substitutes for each other. The FDA wouldn't have a problem with exchanges that make sense. Here's one of their examples: "Try a change for breakfast. A serving of this cereal has __% less fat than a serving of Danish pastry." Both of these items could be considered breakfast foods (although I would hope you'd go for the cereal!).

Health Claims

Descriptive Halos

Nowadays we are bombarded by health claims. Perhaps you don't even realize that you're surrounded by messages appearing on posters and store displays, in magazines, newspapers, and online advertisements, and from friends, family, co-workers, and health professionals. Numerous studies have shown that when a food is given a descriptive halo, it is more likely that people will expect the food to be beneficial to their health, and therefore purchase it. For example, if a bag of pretzels were labeled as a "good source of whole grains," they would be snatched off the shelf faster than a bag that just said "pretzels." Even if the first bag was higher in sodium, it might be chosen because of the grain claim. Dr. Brian Wansink of Cornell's Food and Brand Lab explains that these labels have a dramatic impact because "they allow consumers to concentrate more on their feelings and on the taste of the foods and the sensory nature of the products." Descriptive names are derived from "food-related associations that tie into relevant places, memories, or descriptive adjectives." Trans-fat-free fries, baked chips, and organic candy are all surrounded by health halos, publicizing a possible positive element of the food while underplaying (or ignoring) the negative characteristics. Health halos are far from angelic, though, so read on to uncover the true meaning of the words on your food package.

Claims for certain relationships between a nutrient or a food and the risk of a disease or healthrelated condition are now allowed. They can be made in several ways: through third-party references (such as the American Heart Association), statements, symbols (such as a heart), and vignettes or descriptions. Whatever the case, the claim must meet the requirements for authorized health claims. For example, claims cannot state the specific impact the food will have on your state of health, and they can only use "may" or "might" in discussing the nutrient or food-disease relationship. They must state that other factors play a role in that disease, as controlling disease depends upon a healthy diet in general, not just one food.

The claims also must be written so that consumers can understand the relationship between the nutrient and the disease and the nutrient's importance in an overall daily diet. Translating the above information, an appropriate health claim would be displayed as: "While many factors affect heart disease, diets low in saturated fat and cholesterol *may* reduce the risk of this disease." Manufacturers cannot say, "Consuming this product *will* enable you to lower your cholesterol level *by 15 percent*."

Fast Fact

Trans-fat-free fries and organic candy may be surrounded by health halos, but they're not exactly health foods. Don't be duped by descriptive names that make foods sound better than they really are!

Authorized Health Claims

Scientists have helped us to draw strong associations between food and its benefits in controlling or preventing disease; to this effect the FDA has permitted the following ten nutrient-disease relationship claims to appear on your food labels as long as the manufacturers follow these rules:

1. Calcium and Osteoporosis

To carry a claim which links the calcium content of the food to the prevention of osteoporosis, a food must contain 20 percent or more of the Daily Value for calcium (200 mg) per serving, have a calcium content that equals or exceeds the food's content of phosphorus, and contain a form of calcium that can be readily absorbed and used by the body. The claim must name the target group most in need of adequate calcium intake and also state the need for exercise and a healthy diet. (This is important so people don't think that osteoporosis will be prevented or cured by just eating that one particular food.)

A product that contains 40 percent or more of the Daily Value for calcium must state on the label that a total dietary intake greater than 200 percent of the Daily Value for calcium (that is, 2,000 mg or more) has no further known benefit. (As with most nutrients, although calcium is an important mineral that we often don't get enough of, an intake of 2,500 mg or more of calcium per day generally is not recommended. I mention this because many foods are fortified with calcium, so if you're also taking supplements, you should be careful not to take too much.)

2. Dietary Sugar Alcohols and Dental Caries (Cavities)

This claim regarding the connection between sugar alcohols and dental caries applies to food products such as candy or gum containing the sugar alcohols xylitol, sorbitol, mannitol, maltitol, isomalt, lactitol, hydrogenated starch hydrolysates, hydrogenated glucose syrups, or a combination of any of these. These sugar alcohols or, polyols, do not promote tooth decay (cavities) because bacteria in the mouth cannot easily change polyols to acids that can damage teeth. Besides the food ingredient's relationship to dental caries (cavities), the claim also must state that frequent betweenmeal consumption of foods high in sugars and starches promotes tooth decay. A shortened claim is allowed on food packages with less than fifteen square inches of labeling surface area, such as a package of gum.

3. Fat and Cancer

To carry this claim relating fat and cancer, a food must meet the nutrient content claim requirements for "low-fat" or, if fish and game meats, for "extra-lean."

4. Fiber-Containing Grain Products, Fruits, and Vegetables and Cancer

To carry this claim that associates fiber-rich grain products, fruits, and vegetables with cancer, a food must be or must contain a grain product, fruit, or vegetable and meet the nutrient content claim requirements for "low-fat," and, without fortification, be a "good source" of dietary fiber.

Remember, a high-fiber food has 5 grams or more of fiber per serving and a good source of fiber is one that provides 2.5 to 4.9 grams per serving.

5. Folic Acid and Neural Tube Defects

This claim is allowed on dietary supplements that contain sufficient folate and on conventional foods that are naturally good sources of folate, as long as they do not provide more than 100 percent of the Daily Value for vitamin A as retinol or preformed vitamin A or vitamin D. A sample claim is

"healthful diets with adequate folate may reduce a woman's risk of having a child with a brain or spinal cord defect."

6. Fruits and Vegetables and Cancer

This claim connecting fruits and vegetables with cancer prevention may be made for produce that meets the nutrient content claim requirements for "low-fat" and that, without fortification, for "good source" of at least one of the following: dietary fiber or vitamins A or C. This claim relates to diets low in fat and rich in fruits and vegetables (and thus vitamins A and C and dietary fiber) to reduce cancer risk. The FDA authorized this claim in place of an antioxidant vitamin and cancer claim.

7. Fruits, Vegetables, and Grain Products That Contain Fiber and Risk of Coronary Heart Disease

To carry this claim linking the reduction of heart disease risks and certain beneficial foods, a food must be or must contain fruits, vegetables, and grain products. It also must meet the nutrient content claim requirements for "low saturated fat," "low-cholesterol," and "low-fat" and contain, without fortification, at least 0.6 gram soluble fiber per serving.

8. Saturated Fat and Cholesterol and Coronary Heart Disease

This claim mentioning the link between reduced risk of cardiovascular disease and lower saturated fat and cholesterol intakes may be used if the food meets the definitions for the nutrient content claim "low saturated fat," "low-cholesterol," and "low-fat," or, if fish and game meats, for "extralean."

9. Sodium and Hypertension (High Blood Pressure)

To carry this claim relating sodium intake and hypertension, a food must meet the nutrient content claim requirements for "low-sodium" (140 mg or less per serving).

10. Soluble Fiber Heart Disease

This claim must state that the fiber from certain foods, such as whole oats and psyllium seed husk must also need to be part of a diet low in saturated fat and cholesterol, and the food must provide sufficient soluble fiber to be associated with the ability to reduce heart disease. The amount of soluble fiber in a serving of the food must be listed on the Nutrition Facts Panel. (Learn more about soluble fiber's role in preventing heart disease in Chapter 9.)

Qualified Health Claims

Qualified health claims are those based on potential evidence for the relationship between a food or supplement and a reduced risk of disease. Because the evidence is not well enough established to meet the significant scientific agreement standard, this type of claim must include qualifying language to indicate that the evidence supporting the claim is limited. This disclaimer is to prevent consumers from being misled about the level of support for the claim or other important facts, which could be, for example, conditions of use that are necessary to get the risk reduction benefit. Qualified health claims are considered under the FDA's exercise of enforcement discretion, but they are not authorized by them by regulation.

Some examples of qualified health claims include connections between:
- Omega-3 fatty acids and heart disease
- Calcium supplements and hypertension (high blood pressure)
- Selenium and the risk of certain cancers
- Walnuts and the risk of coronary heart disease

Structure/Function Claims

Structure/function claims describe how a nutrient or substance within the food affects the structure or function of the human body. Interestingly, claims such as these can be made *without* FDA review or authorization before use, but they must be truthful and not misleading and the claims must derive from the nutritional value of the product. This is where things get dicey. This means the *manufacturer* is responsible for conveying accurate information, but the consumer very often is the party that has to be able to comparison shop and resist tantalizing claims.

Here's a scenario one of my patients described to me: While shopping for a bottle of olive oil, he found himself feeling inundated by the vast array of brands and types of this golden liquid. He narrowed down his choices to those that claimed they contained "no cholesterol," but what he didn't know is that no matter which brand he purchased, it would be cholesterol-free, as olive oil never contains cholesterol! For the manufacturer, the goal was accomplished and their product was selected over another that would have been just as good (and perhaps even less expensive).

Other examples of structure/function claims might include the role calcium (nutrient) plays in building strong bones (affects the structure of your body). The claim might read, "calcium builds strong bones." Another instance would show how a substance may act to maintain structure or function, like "fiber maintains bowel regularity." Claims may not, however, specifically link the relationship of a substance to a disease or health-related condition, so, for instance, a label cannot claim, "calcium cures osteoporosis" or "fiber relieves constipation." Those statements would imply an effect on the signs and symptoms of a disease.

Claims: What's Okay to Say?

Using the almond as an example, let me take you through some claims and highlight which are allowed and which would not be acceptable.

First, some background information: Numerous studies have shown that almonds play a role in reducing the risk of heart disease by lowering total cholesterol and low-density lipoprotein (LDL, also known as "bad" cholesterol). In addition to lowering blood lipids, almonds have been found to reduce inflammation, assist in weight management, and hold antioxidant properties. Let's go through the types of claims that could be made about almonds, and which can or can't be used legally:

Nutrient Content Claim: "Almonds are an excellent source of vitamin E." {The claim cannot state, "Almonds are high in vitamin E."}

Structure/Function Claim: "Almonds may help to maintain cholesterol levels that are already within the normal range." {The claim cannot state, "Almonds may help lower cholesterol levels" because legally, the claim cannot imply that almonds could have an effect on a specific disease, in spite of the wealth of scientific evidence supporting such a claim.}

Qualified Health Claim: "Scientific evidence suggests but does not prove that eating 1.5 ounces of most nuts as part of a diet low in saturated fat and cholesterol may reduce your risk of heart disease." {Again, the claim cannot state, "Almonds help lower cholesterol levels."}

Unqualified Health Claim: Here are a few acceptable unqualified health claims for almonds: "Almonds may reduce your risk of heart disease when eaten as part of a low saturated fat and cholesterol diet." "Almonds may reduce your cholesterol as part of a diet low in saturated fat and cholesterol." "Almonds may help maintain a healthy digestive tract." "Almonds may help maintain a healthy cardiovascular system."

Before you run to the supermarket with your cell phone, ready to report misleading declarations to the FDA, here's some more claim information to be on the lookout for. Karen C. Duester, MS, RD, Regulatory Specialist/President of Food Consulting Company, a group that assists manufacturers in developing Nutrition Facts Panels (NFP) for their products, highlighted the following three examples of what manufacturers are not supposed to put on their packages.

Have you seen any of these misleading labels in your supermarket?

You cannot say: "CONTAINS 100 CALORIES." This is a nutrient content claim (the word "contains" makes it so). According to the FDA's definition, "contains" means 10 percent or more DV per serving, and since there is no DV for calories, this is not allowed.

You can say: "100-CALORIE PACK." It's simply a repeat of the information from the NFP— it does not characterize the level as high or low.

You cannot say: "ZERO TRANS FAT PER SERVING." This is a nutrient content claim (the word "zero" makes it so). In the case of trans fat, zero means less than 0.5 gram per serving (same as "no" or "free"), but since there is no DV for trans fats, we cannot have trans fat claims of any type—just quantitative factual statements.

You can say: "0 GRAMS TRANS FAT PER SERVING." You can use the number "0" (rather than the word "zero") because it is replicating the information on the NFP.

You cannot say: "ONLY 3 GRAMS CARB PER SERVING." The word "only" would make this a nutrient content claim. By implication, the word "only" characterizes the carbohydrate content as "low," and the regulations specifically disallow low-carbohydrate claims.

You can say: "3 GRAMS

Chapter 7

Tricky Terms: The Most Manipulative Maneuvers Food Manufacturers Use to Get You to Buy Their Food

Too Good to Be True?

If I were to cite specific examples of how labels can be misconstrued, my book would be too heavy for you to lift! Instead, I'd like to highlight some of the terms that my patients get most perplexed about and some of the products that are brought to my attention because of misleading or confusing information that's displayed on the label (or in the media).

When you're shopping, keep your eyes open for the following ingredients and claims —some of them are legit, but others have health halos beyond which they deserve and belong in the hall of shame.

Here is my hit list:

Agave Syrup

Agave syrup is produced from sap of a plant that has been traditionally used in Mexico. It has become wildly popular, appearing in products ranging from cereal to soda, with the belief that it's a *healthy* sweetener. It is a natural sweetener and has a lower glycemic index than sugar (meaning it doesn't cause as great a surge in blood sugar levels). But before you stock up on agave, notice that it is slightly higher in calories than table sugar, at 20 calories per teaspoon, while sugar has 16 calories. It is sweeter than sugar, though, so you might use less agave than your usual table-top sweet stuff. Just so you're aware, less is best.

Brown Sugar

Brown sugar is refined white sugar that has molasses added to it. Molasses is the syrup that is left over after sugar is processed. The addition of molasses makes brown sugar moister than refined white sugar, but it *doesn't* make it a health food. You will find different types of brown sugar in the supermarket; light brown sugar contains about 3.5 percent molasses, while dark brown sugar contains about 6.5 percent molasses.

Cane Juice

Although the various types of cane juice you'll find on food labels sound earthier than just plain old sugar, it's all the same sweet stuff. In fact, the FDA published a nonbinding recommendation for food companies to stop using the term "evaporated cane juice" because it is confusing for consumers. This labeling suggestion is not mandatory, so for now, look for terms such as cane juice crystals, dehydrated cane juice crystals, unrefined cane juice crystals, raw cane crystals, washed cane juice crystals, unbleached evaporated sugar cane juice crystals, crystallized cane juice, and organic dehydrated cane juice.

Fat-Free

I remember the fat-free craze, when avoiding fat was like avoiding the plague. The words "fat-free" exploded on hundreds of products, including fat-free fat to spread on your fat-free muffins. Yes, those were the 600-calorie muffins, overloaded with sugar but certainly fat-free. Looks like someone forgot to tell us that it's not just watching fat that's needed to fight the battle of the bulge; rather it's all about reducing a little bit of everything. But fat-free foods, and their accompanying labels, continue to attract carb lovers, and our country's rate of obesity continues to climb. Studies have shown that consuming fat-free products can lead to overeating because these foods are less satiating and they provide the illusion of being free of calories and good for you. I'd suggest having a smaller portion of something that may be a little higher in calories, but also ranks higher on the taste scale, such as a small portion of part-skim or even regular cheese versus a block of fat-free cheese. (I call this "low light–soft music food" …something that may be richer, but it's worth appreciating, but in a smaller quantity).

Free-Range or Free-Roaming

Free-range and free-roaming are methods of farming husbandry where the animals are allowed to "roam freely" instead of being contained in any manner. You'll see this label stamped on eggs and on packages of meat and poultry. Farmers may do this to achieve Humane Certification, but these products also command higher prices. The problem is that there is no regulation imposed regarding whether the animals actually spend a good part of their lives outdoors or the amount space the birds have, and therefore this term may be misleading. Free range may mean that a hen has access through only a "pop hole" and not full-body access to roam freely outside. The rule for the label is only that outdoor access is made available for "an undetermined period each day," which is vague at best.

You can check an egg carton for a "Certified Humane®" label from the Humane Farm Animal Care (HFAC) that does have strict definitions. HFAC's Certified Humane® "Free Range" requires birds to have 2 square feet each, whereas HFAC's Certified Humane® "Pasture Raised" requirement is 108 square feet per bird.

Functional Foods

Functional foods are a hot trend in the food industry, and although there is no formal definition for this term, it generally refers to foods or dietary components that may possess health benefits beyond the basic function of providing nutrients. Some foods naturally have these benefits, such as whole grains and fruits and vegetables, while other foods are being developed to contain beneficial components, like yogurt containing added fiber. There are many reasons for this fueled interest in the connection between diet and health, which includes both credible advances in science and technology and incredible claims about how these foods are considered to be a cure-all to any ailment.

Although credible scientific research about a powerhouse of nutrients can be exciting, it can also open to the door to misleading claims and advertisements well beyond the health claims now permitted to be identified by the FDA. Claims related to the cholesterol-lowering ability of oats or the bone-building benefits of calcium-enriched foods have been condoned, as reflected on food labels and in related laws. Other claims, including the potential benefits of vitamins added to a sugary drink, need to be scrutinized. A potential problem with fortified foods is that they create a situation in which it's possible to overconsume particular nutrients. For example, if someone is taking a multivitamin/mineral supplement providing 100 percent of their requirement for vitamin A, and they drink several bottles of vitamin A–enhanced beverages throughout the day, this practice would become harmful rather than helpful.

Although many fortified, enriched, and enhanced foods carry great benefits, it's always preferable to go for foods that provide a natural benefit. It's better to get your omega-3s from fish than potato chips and vitamin C from a fruit than an energy bar. Eating a variety of foods will help you "function" best.

High-Fiber

Fiber has been popping up in places it's never been before, in products ranging from ice cream and yogurt to baked goods. Even foods loaded with sugar can appear more valuable because of an ingredient called polydextrose, a substance used as a fiber supplement that is synthesized from glucose and sorbitol, a sugar alcohol (sugar substitute) found in "sugar-free" products like diet candies, chewing gum, and frozen desserts. Sorbitol has a laxative effect, causing diarrhea and gastrointestinal upset, so proceed with caution when using it. Polydextrose, along with other fiber additives like inulin (derived from chicory root) and maltodextrin (a filler produced from cornstarch), have recently been allowed by FDA approval, to attract those who would normally avoid fiber to welcome it. These fiber additives serve as bulking agents and are listed as and count toward the dietary fiber on the Nutrition Facts Panel. Although these fibers can be beneficial, they may not be as effective as the natural fiber within foods (i.e., the cholesterol-lowering ability of oats as opposed to any of the above fibers added to yogurt). Check the ingredient list to see which fiber you're actually getting.

This is not to say that these fibers are necessarily harmful, though experts don't know for sure if the benefits of high-fiber foods like beans, whole grains, and fruits and vegetables come from the natural fiber itself or from the rich nutrients they contain that work in concert with each other.

Fast Fact

When finding fiber for your diet, be aware that not all fibers are alike. Fibers from polydextrose, inulin, and maltodextrin may count toward your total fiber for the day but may not have the same benefits as those derived from naturally high-fiber foods like beans, whole grains, and fruits and vegetables. These foods are filled with vitamins, minerals, and powerful antioxidants that work in concert with each other.

Hormone-Free or No Hormones (on Milk Cartons)

The FDA has banned the use of claims such as "no hormones" or "hormone-free" on milk cartons because all milk contains naturally occurring hormones. This term was used to make the product look more attractive. There is some debate in the dairy and milk industry about non-organic dairy cows being injected with added, genetically-engineered hormones to increase milk production. This practice was approved by the FDA in 1993 and still considered safe for human consumption, but there is some concern about the effect on human and animal health.

Light

A perfect example of how this term can be confusing is in "light" spreads that contain less fat than typical butter or margarine. Although they are lower in fat content than their full-fat counterparts, they can still be loaded with fat, so use them sparingly. "Light" olive oil, for example, has the same calories as a thick, rich, dark olive oil – it's just lighter in color and flavor.

Local

What does local mean to you? Does it define a food that's grown in your own backyard, your own community, your own city, your own state, or your own region of your own country? Unlike the word "organic," which represents specific criteria for growing/handling/labeling/inspecting such foods, the concept of "local" eating means different things to different people and has no standard definition. The closest description of this word was characterized in 2005 when the term "locavore" was coined by food writer Jessica Prentice for World Environment Day to promote the practice of eating a diet based on food harvested from within an area most commonly bound by a hundred-mile radius. Local also means supporting the use of small farms, consuming foods in season, and eating in a more ecologically sound fashion.

The bottom line on local foods is that they may taste better, fruits and vegetables have a longer period to ripen, and they can be seasonal (and thereby cost less), reduce the risk of contamination (less distance to travel), and support local providers. Foods that are local may be loaded with pesticides, so don't assume otherwise.

In some cases, you may want to ask your store manager where his or her food comes from, and even request that their store purchase food from local vendors. Even better, find a local farmer's market so you can ask the farmers directly where the food is grown!

Low-Impact Carbs, Net Carbs

Early in 2005, not only were there low-carb products in the supermarkets, but there were low-carb aisles in these stores, similarly to how there are now gluten free aisles. Advocates of high-protein diets rejoiced as they loaded up their shopping carts with scores of snacks that had the words "lowimpact carbs" and "net carbs" sprawled across their packaging. These were terms we hadn't heard before this craze—what did they mean? Well, if you looked to the FDA for an answer, you would have been disappointed. This carb lingo was *never* defined or approved by the FDA.

It didn't take a genius to figure out that if you saw a label that displayed, "only 2 grams net carbs" on the front, and the product's Nutrition Facts Panel showed that it had 25 grams of carbohydrate, that something was wrong with the picture. The manufacturer mislead you into believing that this creation would not have any "impact" on your blood sugar (or your weight for that matter) because they deducted the amount of fiber and sugar alcohol the item contained from the total amount of carbohydrates. What they didn't want you to know, however, was that some sugar alcohols have almost as much countable carbohydrate as sugar, and you cannot simply deduct them. In fact, the way to calculate sugar alcohols is by including half of the number of grams displayed on the Nutrition Facts Panel in the number of total carbs. The fiber content of your food should not be discounted if it contains less than 5 grams of carbohydrate.

The good news is that you will see fewer of these labels around because the public is finally waking up to the fact that most of these products were just sugary candy labeled differently, and that they caused their blood sugar levels and weight to go up instead of down after eating them.

Made with Real Fruit

When it comes to juice, be sure that the product you're buying is 100 percent fruit juice. Don't be fooled by labels that call themselves a "juice beverage," "juice cocktail," or "juice drink." These products are a combo of water, sugar, and perhaps some fruit juice, but don't expect much in nutritional value. Be sure to check the ingredient list to make sure the beverage isn't pumped full of cane juice and other sweeteners. You can also check the percent Daily Value listed on the Nutrition Facts Panel. Compare one juice to another to determine which one is worth your money.

This term is often displayed on a lovely package that looks wholesome and pure. Expect to see earth-tone colors and maybe even a picture of a farm in the background. I caution you to look beyond the cozy label, because the FDA has still not set a definition for the word "natural." Moreover, there's no real consistency among manufacturers regarding this term. A review from Mintel Global's new products database shows that in 2008, food and drink claims classified as "natural" were the most frequently featured around the globe, appearing on 23 percent of new products. Here in America, the numbers made an even greater impact, with one-third of new products carrying the "all natural" claim.

This term is "supposed to" convey that the product has no artificial ingredients or intentional additives, but you'll find many of these "natural" foods filled with sugar, fat, and preservatives. According to the FDA, the words "natural flavorings" refer to those that are "derived from a spice, fruit or fruit juice, edible yeast, herb, bark, bud, root, leaf or similar plant material, meat, seafood, poultry, egg, dairy product...whose significant function in food is flavoring rather than nutritional." When the word "natural" is applied to meat or poultry, it generally means the product contains no artificial flavoring, colors, chemical preservatives, or synthetic ingredients. In 2009, the USDA announced its intention to clear up this "natural" progression of confusion through an Advanced Notice of Proposed Rulemaking. The intent is to coordinate both their FSIS and Agricultural Marketing Service's (AMS) definitions of "natural" and "naturally raised." At this point, both of these terms are used voluntarily. It's a step in the right direction. Perhaps clarity in this arena will lead to a change in when and how manufacturers will be allowed to display a "natural" food label, and hopefully it will help consumers distinguish which products are healthiest.

90% Fat-Free

Don't be tricked by the promotion of a food claiming to contain a low percentage of fat. These percentages are based upon the weight of a food. So, for example, a label marked "90% fat-free" might lead you to believe that out of 100 calories, only 10 of them come from fat. This isn't true. It really means that 90 percent of the food is fat-free by weight, so if a food weighs 100 grams, 10 grams (90 calories) will come from fat.

The Nutrition Facts Panel will help you to determine just how much fat your food truly contains by checking the grams of fat. Milk is a good example of this confusing claim. Whole milk contains 3.5 percent fat (3.5 grams of fat per 100 ml). Although this sounds like a pretty low number, when you check the label, you'll find that whole milk contains 8 grams of fat per 8-ounce cup. That's like having a cup of skim milk with almost two pats of butter melted in it. (One pat of butter has 5 grams of fat.) When choosing milk, stick with skim (fat-free) or 1 percent fat types to reap the benefits without the fat.

No-Sugar-Added

This label means that no sugars were added during processing. The product may not contain any "added" sugar, *like poured out of the sugar bowl sugar*, but it can contain "natural" (and we already know how we can't trust this word) sugar. Natural sugars are found in fruit juice concentrates, such as pear nectar, or fruit. Gram for gram, they contain the same amount of sweetness as ordinary sugar and the same calories.

Conversely, don't assume that the amount of sugar on a label means that sugar has been added. A good example of this is the sugar content of milk. Some of my patients come to me thinking that every gram of sugar in every food should be avoided. This is not true for most natural sugars. Milk sugar, or lactose, is accompanied by a host of nine other important nutrients, including protein, calcium, phosphorous, potassium, vitamins A, D, and B_{12}, riboflavin, and niacin. If you need to control your blood sugar, as in the case with diabetes, you may tolerate milk very well because the protein in milk might produce a buffered effect from the carbohydrate (natural sugar) within, thus slowing down the way the carbohydrate is absorbed in your body. To be certain you know where your sugar is coming from, be sure to check the list of ingredients. If you see sugar or high-fructose corn syrup listed early on in the list, you're probably getting more refined sugar "added" to the product than you contemplated.

Good news is that as of January, 2020, the Nutrition Facts Panel has an "added sugar" row underneath the "sugars" row now on the Nutrition Facts Panel to hopefully clear up the confusion surrounding added sugars.

Plus

This term is often used on foods that are fortified with vitamins, minerals, calcium, and a host of other nutrients. The good news is that these sorts of claims fell 20 percent in 2008 according to Mintel Global's new products database, but they still appeared on one in twenty new products launched worldwide. Less use of this word is a "plus" because we should be eating more whole foods that are naturally rich in nutrients instead of those pumped up with added ingredients.

Serving Size

Although this is not a deceptive term, I couldn't help but mention it in this chapter, because this one really pushes my buttons. By manipulating and shrinking the serving sizes of their products, manufacturers can twist reality, showing shockingly low calories, low sugar, and low fat values. For example, "1 cookie" may be listed on the Nutrition Facts Panel as a serving size, but when was the last time you ate just one cookie? This conundrum will hopefully be cleared up as the regulations suggested by the FDA for the new Nutrition Facts Panel (coming soon in 2018) encouraged food manufacturers to make serving sizes more realistic so consumers can easily understand the nutrition content of their food.

Sugar-Free

To make sure that a product doesn't derive most of its carbohydrate content from sugar, check the ingredient listing for words that are sources of sugar, like corn syrup, glucose, sucrose, fructose, maltose, dextrose, honey, high-fructose corn syrup, and molasses. "Sugar-free" is not synonymous with calorie-free, nor is it necessarily low calorie. A sugar-free chocolate bar could still be laden with fat and sodium. Calories in such products can also get a boost from other starches and artificial sweeteners and sugar alcohols such as sorbitol, mannitol, and xylitol. These substances, in small amounts, can be enjoyed without having an effect on blood sugar levels, but when taken in excess can cause numbers to climb. In addition, sugar alcohols can cause gas and diarrhea, so you may want to cut back on portions to curtail gastrointestinal distress.

Sustainable

This is a hot word on so many lips...even though many people don't even know what it means. Sustainability includes buying food as close to home as possible and it involves food production methods that respect workers, provide fair wages to farmers, support farming communities, do not harm the environment, and that are healthy and are humane to animals. Buying *local* food (see above), however, does not guarantee that it is sustainably produced. Pesticides, chemical fertilizers, factory farming, hormone use, and non-therapeutic use of antibiotics can all be involved in local food production.

Wheat Bread

Just because you just chose a dark brown bread from the supermarket doesn't necessarily mean you are getting a product bursting with fiber or whole grains. The color could be the result of molasses or caramel coloring. When selecting bread, be sure the first ingredient is 100 percent whole wheat or a whole grain.

Almost all flour comes from wheat and can be called "wheat flour," even if it is processed, bleached, and stripped of important nutrients. Products with "wheat" in their name may not necessarily be carrying the whole-grain goodness even if the label shows a stalk of wheat swaying in the wind. Be sure to check your ingredient list to see which grains are being used in the product. The words "whole grain" or "100% whole wheat" should be mentioned first on this list to be sure you're getting the nutrient-rich carbohydrate you're paying for. Take note, however, that even if bread is not 100 percent whole wheat, it can still be nutritious. Enriched breads made from oats, sprouted wheat, cracked wheat, and wheat bran can be a part of a healthy diet.

0 Grams Trans Fat

When reading labels, you can find trans fats listed as "hydrogenated" or "partially hydrogenated" fats. In 2006, food manufacturers were required by the Food and Drug Administration to list the trans fat contents of all food on the Nutrition Facts Panel. But buyer beware! There was a loophole: The FDA allowed food manufacturers to label any product that has less than a gram of trans fat per serving as "0 grams trans fats." That means you could be getting 0.49 gram of trans fat in a single serving and not know it. Does 0.40 equal 0? Not exactly. This may not seem like a big deal, but if you couple this with unrealistic serving sizes, the likelihood is that you could be consuming a lot more trans fat than you bargained for. Portion distortion problems are common, as reflected in improbable serving sizes listed on packages that do not reveal the larger quantities we actually ingest.

But there's good news too. In 2015, the FDA announced a ban on the inclusion of artificial trans fat in the food supply in America. This requires food manufacturers to remove partially hydrogenated oils from their products over the next couple of years.

For now, the only way to tell if an item truly has 0 grams of trans fat is to look through the ingredient list. If any of the ingredients are either hydrogenated or partially hydrogenated fat, then bingo…trans fats are in that product.

Chapter 8

Deciphering the Diseases

I have a patient who said to me, "I have so many different people to shop for: My husband has diabetes and hypertension, my cholesterol is high and I have osteoporosis, I shop for my elderly mom who is recovering from chemotherapy, and then I have to buy the foods my kids like, too. How do I meet everyone's needs without spending a fortune and taking hours to go through the supermarket?"

Sadly, statistics show that if you can relate to the situation above, you are not alone. It is certainly a challenge to shop and cook properly for all the members of your family, and while various health concerns can require different diets, the foundation of what each person needs to eat rests upon very similar eating plans.

This chapter is not meant to take the place of a visit with a doctor or registered dietitian. The fact is that a lot of us, and the people we love, face medical challenges that can be improved, or perhaps even prevented, through some basic modifications in diet. I'm hoping that the following information will shed light on what you may need to pay closer attention to if you have any of the medical conditions mentioned below. Although the way we react to different foods and ingredients may vary, one thing is for sure: Our health can be directly affected by the food we put (or don't put) in our mouths.

Food Allergies and Food Sensitivities

Having food allergies is a serious medical condition. Many people think that allergy symptoms are limited to some sniffles, itchy eyes, or stomachache, but some food allergies can be life-threatening. For those who are highly allergic, even touching or smelling a particular food could produce a severe reaction.

The Food Allergen Labeling and Consumer Protection Act of 2004 (FALCPA) was enacted to address the labeling of all packaged foods regulated by the FDA. Believe it or not, there are more than 160 foods have been identified to cause food allergies in sensitive individuals, but the "major food allergens" account for 90 percent of all food allergies. Under FALCPA, a "major food allergen" is an ingredient that is one of the following eight foods or food groups or an ingredient that contains protein derived from one of them: milk, egg, fish, crustacean shellfish (including crab, lobster, and shrimp), tree nuts, wheat, peanuts, and soybeans.

Allergens other than the major food allergens are not subject to FALCPA labeling requirements. FALCPA labeling requirements apply to foods that are made with any ingredient, including flavorings, colorings, or incidental additives (e.g., processing aids), that is or contains a major food allergen.

To alert consumers as to which allergen might be within their product, a "contains" statement must appear on the label (e.g., "contains soybeans"). This statement must be placed immediately above the manufacturer, packer, or distributor statement. Furthermore, if a "contains" statement is used on a food label, the statement must include the names of the food sources of all major food allergens used as ingredients in the packaged food. For example, if sodium caseinate, whey, egg yolks, and natural peanut flavor are included on a product's ingredient list, any "contains" statement appearing on the label immediately after or near that statement is required to identify all three sources of the major food allergens present (e.g., "contains milk, eggs, and peanuts") in the same type (print or font) size as that used for the ingredient list.

Other key phrases, such as "may contain nuts," "produced on shared equipment with nuts or peanuts," or "produced in a facility that also processes nuts," must appear on food labels even if the food produced might not contain nuts themselves. These warnings are there to prevent crosscontamination from nuts that may have been contained in other foods being produced and packaged within the same plant and got mixed in accidentally.

The following summary will help lead you through what to look for on labels regarding common food allergies and sensitivities.

Milk Allergy and Lactose Intolerance

Don't confuse a milk allergy with lactose intolerance; the two are quite different. Someone with a milk allergy needs to *avoid* all the foods and ingredients that are listed below. With lactose intolerance, depending on your level of sensitivity, you may need to either eliminate or reduce your intake of foods that contain lactose. Remember that ingredients are listed by weight, so if any of the above items are listed third or fourth, for example, you may be able to tolerate the product better than if the item is listed first.

Recognizing these items is not always easy, as the word "lactose" may not actually appear on the label. There are also hidden sources of lactose in foods that you wouldn't expect to find it in, like hot dogs and salad dressings. Lactose-containing foods include:

- Butter
- Buttermilk
- Cheese
- Chocolate milk
- Cottage cheese
- Cream cheese
- Dry powdered milk
- Evaporated milk
- Half-and-half
- Ice cream
- Ice milk
- Light cream
- Margarine
- Milk
- Milk chocolate
- Milk solids
- Ricotta cheese
- Sherbet
- Shortening
- Sour cream
- Sweetened condensed milk
- Whey
- Whipping cream
- Yogurt

In addition, check the Nutrition Facts Panel and ingredient list for words like:

- Lactate
- Lactic acid
- Lactalbumin
- Casein
- Caseinate

- Lactylate

Gluten Allergy

Celiac disease, a genetic, autoimmune disorder, also referred to as CD, is a digestive disorder in which gluten cannot be tolerated that can affect adults and children. Depending on the severity of the disorder, even a small amount of gluten in the diet can be harmful, producing symptoms including diarrhea, abdominal pain, bloat, nausea, vitamin and mineral deficiencies, chronic fatigue and damage to the small intestine. Gluten is the layman's term for a protein found in all forms of grains derived from wheat, barley, rye, triticale, and in some cases oats. Gluten can be found in cereals, breads, baked goods, desserts, cookies, crackers, baking mixes, flours, grains, pastas, entrees, side dishes, and many other snacks and prepared foods. Those who need to follow a glutenfree diet must always be vigilant about label reading, especially because many manufacturers change their products without notifying the public. Something you might have enjoyed previously may now be unsafe. Other foods that have gluten where you might not suspect its presence are soy sauce, licorice, luncheon meats, and imitation seafood, just to mention a few.

Proceed with caution when it comes to using oats, though several manufacturers are producing pure and uncontaminated oats and oat products grown on dedicated fields and harvested, transported, and processed with dedicated equipment.

For the person who has celiac disease, it may be a challenge to meet your requirements for B vitamins and fiber because many gluten-free foods are not vitamin-enriched and lack thiamin, riboflavin, niacin, iron, and folate [B vitamins]. However, with the growth of gluten sensitivity and the demand for gluten-free products, there has been a trend for companies to enrich their products, making them more nutritionally beneficial.

In 2013, the FDA passed a rule that companies may voluntarily label their products as "gluten free" if they abide by certain regulations. These regulations include that a product is inherently gluten free or does not contain any gluten-containing ingredients, or if gluten is unavoidable, a product contains less than 20 parts per million (ppm) of gluten.

Look for the chart outlining foods that may contain hidden sources of gluten and glutencontaining grains, as well as foods that can be enjoyed safely at the end of this chapter.

Fast Fact

Gluten is the layman's term for a protein found in all forms of grains derived from wheat, barley, rye, triticale, and in many cases, oats. Don't confuse a gluten allergy with an allergy to wheat.

Wheat Allergy

Wheat is a found in a wide variety of products, including breads, pasta, cereal, noodles, prepared foods, baked goods, breaded foods, ice cream, hot dogs, sauces, dressings, food thickeners, hydrolyzed vegetable protein, flavorings, and many more. Check labels carefully. Don't confuse a wheat allergy with an intolerance to gluten: Even though people with celiac disease and people with wheat allergies have similar dietary restrictions—the must avoid all wheat in the diet—celiacs must also avoid other gluten-containing grains like rye and barley. Moreover, celiac disease is an immune disorder that affects the body's ability to process *gluten proteins found in wheat* and some other grains, but is not a *wheat allergy*. Symptoms of those with wheat allergies

68

include asthma, eczema, or, in extreme cases, anaphylaxis. In celiac disease, the gastrointestinal tract generally is what is most affected.

Nut Allergy

If you have a nut allergy, you need to strictly avoid nuts, including peanuts and tree nuts (almonds, Brazil nuts, cashews, chestnuts, filberts, hazelnuts, hickory nuts, macadamia nuts, pecans, pine nuts, pistachios, and walnuts) and food containing nuts and nut oils to prevent a reaction. In some cases, this may be easier said than done, because nuts may be included in products that you would never suspect, like ice cream, salad dressings, cereals, sauces, or cookies. You'd never know that hydrolyzed vegetable (or plant) protein listed on the ingredient list may be derived from peanuts and should be passed up.

Label reading is essential if you have a nut allergy, and don't assume that the product that was nut-free the last time you bought it is still made without nuts today. Check the ingredient list on every product you buy and/or check with the manufacturer before consuming any food in question. It's also important to look for the "contains" statement or similar warning statements like "may contain nuts," as described above, to prevent cross-contamination.

If you have been carefully tested and are certain that you are allergic only to peanuts, then you can safely eat tree nuts (almonds, cashews, and hazelnuts) and their nut butters. If you cannot eat any nut butter, then soy nut butter is a delicious alternative, provided you are not allergic to soy. Sunflower butter is higher in fiber and iron than peanut butter, and is safe for people with peanut allergies.

Soy Allergy

If you are allergic to soy, avoid products with the following words on the ingredient list: edamame, hydrolyzed soy protein, miso, natto, shoyu, soy (soy albumin, soy fiber, soy grits, soy beverage, soy nuts, soy sprouts), soya, soybean (curd, granules), soy protein (concentrate, isolate), soy sauce, tamari, tempeh, tofu, lecithin, monodiglyceride, monosodium glutamate (MSG), vegetable oil, vitamin E, natural flavoring, vegetable broth, vegetable gum and vegetable starch, hydrolyzed vegetable protein, and textured vegetable protein (TVP). Some people who are soy-allergic may be able to consume soybean oil and soy lecithin, but check with your doctor before eating any foods that may be questionable.

Egg Allergy

Eggs are the masters of disguise. They can be hidden in mayonnaise, meringue, baked goods, cake mixes, batters, sauces, frosting, processed meat, meatloaf, meatballs, pudding, salad dressing, noodles, commercial egg substitutes, gourmet coffee drinks, and marshmallows, just to name a few. Here are some other names for eggs that may appear on your ingredient list: albumin, albuminate, globulin, lecithin, livetin, lysozyme, vitellin, and words that begin with ova or ovo (such as ovalbumin or ovoglobulin).

Crustacean Shellfish Allergy

Crab, lobster, shrimp, and ingredients that contain protein derived from crustacean shellfish are major food allergens. Molluscan shellfish, such as oysters, clams, mussels, or scallops, are not major food allergens.

Fish Allergy

All varieties of freshwater fish and seafood should be avoided if you are allergic to fish. Read labels carefully, as fish may be mentioned by name rather than just the word "fish." For example, anchovies rather than fish will most likely be listed in the ingredients in a bottle of Caesar salad dressing.

Diabetes

The Serving Size: Serving sizes are standardized and under the guise of the FDA, but that doesn't mean that they aren't confusing. The standard amount shown on the package is supposed to be *one* "typical" serving. Good news: The updated Nutrition Facts Panels [coming to a package near you in 2018] should reflect more realistic serving sizes. Still, make sure you're eating the serving size listed so that you don't end up eating more calories than your body requires—or counting only half the calories you've consumed if you're watching your daily total.

Type of Carbohydrate: The various forms of carbohydrate (refined/simple, complex, unprocessed, etc.) affect blood glucose levels in different ways, and we as individuals don't all process carbs the same way. It's best to emphasize complex types and whole grains as opposed to refined, simple carbs.

Naturally occurring sugars, such as fructose in fruit and lactose in milk, provide healthy sources of energy, vitamins, carbohydrate, and minerals. Added sugars, on the other hand, are included in foods during processing, in food preparation, or at the table. Food processing is now the greatest contributor of added sugars. Often the added ingredient is high-fructose corn syrup. You will soon be able to easily identify added sugars on the new Nutrition Facts panel as a new category is now required on the updated panels.

In any event, and most important, remember that foods labeled as "sugar-free" or "no added sugar" are not necessarily calorie- or carbohydrate-free. Look at the ingredient list to check where your sugar is coming from, because the word "sugars" on the label does not allow you to distinguish between the two types of sugars.

Sugar Alcohols: These are carbohydrate-based ingredients that are often added to foods to provide a super-sweet taste. Mistakenly, people assume that these products are like artificial sweeteners and have no calories. This is not true at all, but someone forgot to tell this to manufacturers!

So a food label may not list sugar as an ingredient, but the label should state that it has 20 grams of sugar alcohol—that's equal to the calories in about 10 grams of sugar. The reason they provide fewer calories is because they are not completely digested. But that doesn't mean that they can just be ignored. Sometimes they're hard to ignore: these sugar alcohols, or polyols, as they are called, can cause gas, bloating, cramps, or diarrhea as a side effect. The FDA warns you about this with an information statement: "Excess consumption may have a laxative effect," so, yes, consuming these products can be a moving experience.

You can recognize sugar alcohols because they usually end in the letters -ol. Some examples of these ingredients are sorbitol, mannitol, xylitol, lactitol, isomalt, maltitol, and hydrogenated starch hydrolysates (HSH).

Fiber: Fiber is an important nutrient in your diet because it can affect the rate at which food moves through your system, thereby playing a role in controlling your blood sugar. A high-fiber diet will slow the release of glucose into your blood after a meal, as well as improve cholesterol levels and digestion.

To boost your fiber intake, try to choose whole grain breads containing at least 3 grams of fiber per slice. A cereal that's high in fiber contains 5 grams of fiber or more per serving, but if these types of cereals are not usually found on your shopping list, try mixing one of your favorite (less healthy) brands with a high-fiber brand to enhance its value. Other great sources of fiber are beans, vegetables, and whole grains like barley and buckwheat.

Heart Disease/Controlling Cholesterol

Calories: Two-thirds of Americans are taking in too much and putting out too little; we're overweight and underactive. If you're tipping the scales, even weight loss of ten to fifteen pounds can put less pressure on your heart and decrease your risk of future heart disease.

Cholesterol: Cholesterol is manufactured in your liver and is present in foods of animal origin, like meat, poultry, and full-fat dairy products. The amount of cholesterol absorbed from food and type that circulates in the body can determine your level of cardiovascular health. When your doctor checks your blood, he or she will be analyzing for blood lipoproteins (containing lipids and proteins), including high-density lipoprotein (HDL) cholesterol and low-density lipoprotein (LDL) cholesterol—also known as "good" and "bad" cholesterol, respectively. Excessive buildup of LDL cholesterol can cause plaque (fatty deposits) that accumulates in arteries, possibly leading to high blood pressure, heart attack, or stroke. The 2015 *Dietary Guidelines* no longer suggest limiting dietary cholesterol intake to a specific upper limit as in the past. The recent *Guidelines*, however, do recommend limiting dietary cholesterol intake to as little as possible.

Saturated fat: Saturated fat may create even more of a risk of developing heart disease than cholesterol, so when you're reading the Nutrition Facts Panel, don't just glance down at the cholesterol value; check how much saturated fat is in that product, too. NCEP guidelines advise reducing your intake of saturated fats to less than 10 percent of daily caloric intake. That means that if you're trying to lose weight and you are consuming 1,500 calories each day, you should try to limit your intake of saturated fats to a total of 15 grams daily. Keep in mind that this number not only includes the numbers you see reflected on the food label (listed in grams of saturated fat), but it also includes the saturated fat that's present in meat, poultry, eggs, and other products you consume that may not carry a Nutrition Facts Panel.
Trying to limit saturated fat has been judged by some people as unnecessary, with the claims that sat fat is not as harmful for as us previously believed. This is reflected in the fact that coconut oil and its related products are on fire – appearing on supermarket shelves and in our pantries more than ever. But proceed with caution when it comes to saturated fat – just because it may not be as harmful, it doesn't mean that it's beneficial. Other fats, like those in olive oil, avocado or nuts, have been shown to reduce the incidence of heart disease, so perhaps it's best to consume a mix of fats in the diet.

Trans fat: The number next to trans fat on your label should be "0," and even zero could be more that you realize because of a labeling loophole. Even though food companies are required to remove artificial trans fats by June 2018, be sure to check the small print in the ingredients section and avoid "hydrogenated oils."

Sodium: Your diet should be in keeping with the recommended level of 2,300 mg of sodium each day for healthy individuals. The American Heart Association recommends that certain individuals could benefit from limiting their sodium intake to 1,500 mg, but this number would be unrealistic for most of us. Speak with your physician or dietitian to determine an appropriate sodium intake level for you and read labels carefully. Seventy-five percent of the sodium we eat comes from packaged foods with the remainder coming from the salt we shake at the table.

Fiber: Fiber can help cholesterol levels come down if you make the right choices. Foods rich in soluble fiber like oats, beans, barley, and many fruits and vegetables (apples, oranges, and carrots) should make up one-quarter of your total fiber intake for the day. Shoot for 25 to 35 grams of fiber in total, which will also help control blood sugar levels and keeps thing moving smoothly through your digestive tract.

There are times, however, when a diet high in fiber (especially soluble fiber) and low in saturated fat and cholesterol, and a medically safe exercise program may not be enough to keep blood lipids in check. Unless your physician feels that cholesterol-lowering medications may be warranted, you might consider the addition of plant sterols/stanols to your diet. Furthermore, for certain people, it has been found that cholesterol levels can be reduced even more dramatically through a combination of plant sterols/stanols along with medications. As with any medical strategy, you should always check with your health care provider to determine what the best treatment is in your particular case.

Fast Fact

Foods rich in soluble fiber like oats, beans, barley, and many fruits and vegetables (apples, oranges, and carrots) should make up at least one-quarter of the 25 to 30 grams of fiber you should be getting each day.

High Blood Pressure (Hypertension)

Sodium: "Sodium has become the new trans-fat," reports Mintel Global market research firm. Even more than the actual salt shaker at the table, most of the sodium we eat (75 percent) comes from foods that come in packages. Not only are fresh foods like fruits and vegetables better because they are inherently healthier, but they're also foods of choice because they're not highly processed. Although canned vegetables are an excellent source of vitamins and minerals, when it comes to sodium, fresh and frozen foods are best, unless you thoroughly rinse items that are canned. You can decrease the sodium content in canned beans, for example, by rinsing then thoroughly. Opt for low-sodium versions (less than 140 mg per serving) or moderate-sodium (less than 400 mg per serving) types of foods when available.

Serving sizes: Don't be fooled by a low value next to the word sodium before checking the portion size it is referring to where it says "servings per container." Multiply the sodium value by the amount of servings you plan to consume.

Calories: As your body weight increases, your blood pressure could rise: keeping calories in check can control both.

Ingredient list: Be sure to check the ingredient list to spot sodium-containing ingredients like monosodium glutamate (MSG), sodium benzoate, sodium hydroxide, sodium nitrite, sodium propionate, disodium phosphate, and sodium sulfate. Additives such as these are the reason why the number of milligrams of sodium on some products is so high even when the word "salt" doesn't appear on the label.

Fast Fact

Check labels for sodium's close relatives: monosodium glutamate (MSG), sodium benzoate, sodium hydroxide, sodium nitrite, sodium propionate, disodium phosphate, and sodium sulfate.

Osteoporosis

Did you know that your bones are living tissues and they continue to change throughout your life? During childhood and adolescence, bones increase in size and strength and continue to add more mass until peak bone mass is reached. Although this is believed to occur around age thirty, up to 90 percent of peak bone mass is actually acquired by age eighteen in girls and age twenty in boys, which makes these early years a critical time for bone building. This highlights the importance of consuming adequate amounts of calcium and vitamin D throughout infancy, childhood, and adolescence to help delay or avoid bone loss as you age.

Fiber: Excess fiber can bind with calcium and thereby interfere with its absorption. It's rare that we get a surplus of fiber through foods; too much fiber through supplements is possible, though. Follow label instructions or check with your health care provider when considering nonfood supplemental fiber.

Excessive sodium: In addition to raising your blood pressure, sodium can also increase urinary calcium excretion. Remember to check the Nutrition Facts Panel for sodium content of foods, too.

Protein: Urinary excretion of calcium can also be increased by consuming an excessively high amount of protein, so forget the fad diets and help your weight and your bones with a better balanced eating plan. Generally speaking, between 10 and 15 percent of your total calories should come from protein. So, for example, if you consume 2,000 calories per day, that means 200 to 300 calories should come from protein, or about 50 to 75 grams. As a frame of reference, one ounce of protein (like meat, poultry or fish) contains around 7 grams of protein.

Calcium: This is the major component of bones, and therefore is one of the most important dietary factors relating to osteoporosis. The Nutrition Facts Panel (NFP) on your food label will provide the information you'll need to determine how much calcium is in the packaged food you eat. The percent Daily Value for calcium is 1,000 mg, although some of us may need to take in more than that level, depending on age and factors such as whether a person is pregnant or lactating.

Vitamin D: Every superhero needs a sidekick, and in this case, calcium's partner is vitamin D. Vitamin D is so important and a nutrient of concern in America that the new Nutrition Facts Panel will require vitamin D content to be listed on all labels. Vitamin D helps with the absorption of calcium. Your body can make vitamin D when your skin is exposed to sunlight and you can obtain vitamin D from food. Aside from bone health, vitamin D has also been shown to boost immune function and decrease inflammation, which, respectively, are role players in reducing the risks of cancer and heart disease. Very few foods naturally contain vitamin D, but you can find it in the flesh of fatty fish (such as salmon, tuna, and mackerel) and fish liver oils. Foods fortified with vitamin D provide most of this important nutrient in our diet, particularly in milk (100 IU per cup of vitamin D, equivalent to 25 percent of the Daily Value). In the United States, foods allowed to be fortified with vitamin D include cereal flours, some breakfast cereals and related products, milk and products made from milk, and calcium-fortified fruit juices and drinks. In 2010, the recommended daily allowance (RDA) of vitamin D was increased to 600 IU per day for those 1-70 years old, 800 IU per day for pregnant or breastfeeding women and 800 IU per day for those over 71 years old.

Foods and Beverages That May Contain Gluten

Food Category	Food Products	Notes
Meats and alternatives	Deli/luncheon meats, hot dogs, sausage, imitation seafood (such as surimi)	May contain fillers made from wheat. Seasonings may contain hydrolyzed wheat protein, wheat flour, or wheat starch.
	Frozen burgers (meat, poultry, and fish); meatloaf	May contain fillers (wheat flour, wheat starch, bread crumbs) or seasonings (see above).
	Meat substitutes (such as vegetarian burgers, sausage, nuggets)	Often contain hydrolyzed wheat protein, wheat gluten, wheat starch, or barley malt.
	Baked beans	Some are thickened with wheat flour.
	Tempeh	A meat substitute made from fermented soybeans and sometimes other grains such as millet or rice. Often seasoned with soy sauce (made from wheat).
Grains and starches	Rice and corn cereals	May contain barley malt extract or barley malt flavoring.
	Buckwheat flour	Pure buckwheat flour is gluten-free; however, some buckwheat flour may be mixed with wheat flour.
	Buckwheat pasta (soba noodles)	Most soba noodles are a combination of buckwheat flour and wheat flour.
	Seasoned or flavored rice mixes	Seasonings may contain hydrolyzed wheat protein, wheat flour, or wheat starch or have added soy sauce derived from wheat
Milk and dairy	Cheese spreads, cheese sauces (such as nacho), seasoned flavored shredded cheese	May be thickened with wheat flour or wheat starch. Seasonings may contain hydrolyzed wheat protein, wheat flour, or wheat starch.
Snack foods	Seasoned potato chips, taco (corn) chips, nuts, soy nuts	Some brands of plain potato chips contain wheat starch or wheat flour (such as Pringles). Seasoning mixes may contain hydrolyzed wheat protein, wheat flour, or wheat starch.
	Chocolate, chocolate bars	May contain wheat flour or barley malt flavoring.
	Licorice	Regular brands of licorice contain wheat flour. Some brands of gluten-free licorice are available.
Condiments and sauces	Soy sauce	Many brands are a combination of soy and wheat.

	Malt vinegar	Made from malted barley. As this vinegar is only fermented and not distilled, it contains varying levels of gluten.
	Salad dressings	May contain wheat flour, malt vinegar, or soy sauce (made from wheat). Seasonings may contain hydrolyzed wheat protein, wheat flour,
		or wheat starch.
	Specialty prepared mustards	Some brands may contain wheat flour.
Miscellaneous	Cake icing and frostings	May contain wheat flour or wheat starch.
	Baking powder	Most brands contain cornstarch, which is gluten-free. However, some brands may contain wheat starch.
	Cooking sprays	Cooking spray may contain wheat flour or wheat starch.
Beverages	Flavored or herbal teas, flavored coffees	May contain barley malt flavoring. Some specialty coffees may be prepared with a chocolate-chip-type product that contains cookie crumbs.
	Beer, ale, and lager	Made from malted barley. Some brands of gluten-free beer are now available.
	Alcoholic cooler beverages	May contain barley malt.

Source: *Gluten-Free Diet: A Comprehensive Resource Guide*, Revised and Expanded Edition, Shelley Case, RD, Case Nutrition Consulting Inc, 2010, www.glutenfreediet.ca

Part Two

Navigating the Aisles: How to Shop for the Best Foods

Now we're going to walk down the aisle together (how romantic!). I'll help you weigh your options and make the best choices among the vast array of food products on those supermarket shelves. You shouldn't have to be required to be a dietitian, mathematician, or librarian to put the healthy food in your shopping cart, but believe it or not, even nutrition professionals sometimes have a hard time assessing which foods are "best."

I remember that when I got my first job and attended hospital medical rounds with doctors, I was shocked to hear how different their opinions were about treating their patients' illnesses. I had always assumed that there was *one answer* when it came to dealing with a diagnosis, but I soon learned that was not the case. We see a similar story in the supermarket: the question of what's best does not have one simple answer.

As I was researching this book, I asked fellow registered dietitian nutritionists to share their opinions about their top food choices and the standards they use when helping patients improve shopping habits. This time I wasn't surprised that I received many different answers. Many responses suggested relying on the FDA standards I cited earlier in Chapter 3. I relied on these responses as well as my own expertise as a dietitian nutritionist to put together this part of this book, where I will take you into each section of the grocery store and help you choose the healthiest bread, milk, cereal, and so on.

Before we get started, you should know that there's good and bad news about food shopping with me: The bad news is that I won't necessarily tell you which brands to buy. I don't want you to feel that a specific manufacturer's name or the item's price should stand in your way of making an educated decision about whether or not to purchase a product. Although I do have allegiances to certain brands that I enjoy and trust, since new products come to market daily, I tried to provide you with general guidelines without making you feel right or wrong regarding your purchases and personal preferences.

The good news, however, is that the sky's the limit! I will help you assemble a powerhouse of foods without restricting you or telling you what to do. I want you to be able to shop in *any* store, *any*where across the country and know that you will be able to fill your cart with nourishing foods for your entire family. You shouldn't just judge a food by the number, check, or star that it may wear on its label or nearby shelf tag; those symbols and values use different systems to rate foods, often presenting conflicting information. My goal is for you to discover your own favorite products so you can streamline food purchases to fit your own personal needs.

So, let's step through those sliding doors, feel that gust of cold air flowing around your local supermarket, and go shopping!

Chapter 9

Finding Fruits and Visiting Vegetables: The Produce Aisle

During the thirty-something years I have been in the nutrition business, I have never had a patient come to me overweight because they were eating too many fruits and vegetables. These jewels of the nutrition crown are always number one on any list of foods that help avoid heart disease, thwart cancer, aid digestion, ease inflammation, and promote weight loss.

Maybe if you took a closer look at what fruits and vegetable contribute to your diet, you'll spend more time in the produce aisle than any other. Here are just some of the reasons why these foods should take up at least half your plate at each meal and be a part of your snacks:

High fiber: Fruits and vegetables are naturally high in fiber; they don't need to add any, as other products do, to claim that they provide this important nutrient.

Low sodium: Fruits and vegetables that are unprocessed (meaning fresh, not from a can) are either sodium-free or extremely low in sodium.

No cholesterol: Plants do not make cholesterol; thus, any food that comes from a plant is naturally cholesterol-free.

Loads of vitamins, minerals, antioxidants, phytochemicals, and more: There's no food group that has more nutritional value than fruits and vegetables. The array of color displays their range of nutrients provided by Mother Nature's pharmacy. Vitamins A and C, iron, potassium, magnesium, selenium, lycopene, and resveratrol are just a few of the vitamins and minerals provided by fruits and vegetables.

Health links: Countless studies have linked a diet high in fruits and vegetables with a reduced incidence of various diseases, including cancer, heart disease, cataracts, hypertension, diabetes, and arthritis.

Fast Fact

I have never had a patient come to me overweight because they were eating too many fruits and vegetables. You don't have to count every calorie that comes from these foods—just count on them filling you up without them filling you out.

Fruits and vegetables can be found in a variety of forms in the supermarket—fresh, dried, frozen, and canned. Let's explore this food group together.

How to Shop for *Fresh* Fruits and Vegetables

Fresh fruits and vegetables come in all different shapes, sizes, and colors. These beauties are nutrient-rich in their natural state without processing. Fresh fruits and vegetables have a shorter shelf life than dried, frozen, or canned.

Seasonal and Local

Though today's supermarkets make even summer favorites available in winter, for the deepest nutrient value, purchase fresh produce that is in season. Most produce that is bought out of season has traveled anywhere between 1,500 and 2,500 miles to get to you, and produce purchased out of season was picked before it ripened. This affects both the taste and the amount of vitamins and minerals present. From an environmental perspective, produce that has to travel long distances uses valuable resources, such as oil, which harms the environment. For this reason, it is important to try to purchase not only seasonal produce but also produce that is locally grown, which ensures minimal transport time, better taste, higher quality, and the additional benefit of supporting local farmers.

You can't necessarily tell where your produce comes from or how high in quality it is just by looking at it, and shelf tags are not always available to provide you with such information. Believe it or not, the best way to find out which produce in your supermarket is local is to ask. Ask your store manager, or if your supermarket employs a registered dietitian nutritionist, ask her or him. You can also look online by searching www.localharvest.org or www.eatwellguide.org to find farmers' markets, family farms, and other sources of sustainably grown food in your area. One of my favorite sites, www.epicurious.com, displays an interactive seasonal ingredient map that helps you to find what's fresh in your area, plus ingredient descriptions, shopping guides, recipes, and tips.

A Palate of Color
Try to pick as many bright, deeply colored types of produce, including red (tomatoes, strawberries), orange (sweet potatoes, carrots), green (broccoli, kale), yellow (squash, peppers), and white (onions, garlic).

Organic Fruits and Vegetables
If we're supposed to be consuming about two cups of fruit and 2 ½-3 cups of vegetables each day, then whether we are eating organic or not could make a big difference in what we're putting into our bodies.

Organic doesn't only refer to the food itself—it's also about how the food was produced. It will be your personal decision whether purchasing organic foods is worth the price. If you're considering making the switch, perhaps start with choosing organic over conventional types of the "dirty dozen" fruits and vegetables, which weigh in with greater pesticide levels, but save your money on the "clean fifteen."

The Dirty Dozen
According to the Environmental Working Group (EWG), consumers can reduce their pesticide exposure by 80 percent by avoiding the most contaminated fruits and vegetables. Based on statistical analysis of testing conducted by the USDA and the FDA, EWG has been publishing these yearly guides referring to the most pesticide-contaminated foods, even after they are washed properly. The 2017 "Dirty Dozen" list according to the EWG includes:

- Apples
- Bell peppers
- Cherries
- Celery
- Grapes
- Greens: lettuce, spinach
- Nectarines
- Peaches
- Pears
- Potatoes
- Strawberries
- Tomatoes

On the other hand, the "clean 15" may not warrant a switch to organic, which also makes purchasing these foods easier on your wallet. (And yes, even though math is not my specialty, I know this list contains more than fifteen items!)

The Clean 15

- Asparagus
- Avocados
- Broccoli
- Cabbage
- Cantaloupe
- Cauliflower
- Corn
- Eggplant
- Garlic
- Grapefruit
- Honeydew melon
- Kiwis
- Mangos
- Onions
- Papaya
- Pineapple
- Shelling peas

Plants Rule

I'd like you to hear this message as if I'm holding a megaphone: IT'S BETTER TO EAT FRUITS AND VEGETABLES THAT MAY CONTAIN PESTICIDES THAN NOT TO EAT FRUITS AND VEGETABLES AT ALL.

Sorry to shout . . . but you don't need a food label to tell you that eating fruits and vegetables is the key to good health, optimal weight, and the best food choices.

Country of Origin Labeling (COOL) Labeling

Although our consumption of fruits and vegetables has increased, as a country we are nowhere near the 5 to 10 servings per day recommended by the Centers for Disease Control and Prevention. Because of the seasonality of domestic produce supplies and the perceived belief that fresh produce is best, imports are often relied upon. COOL labeling will let you know how far your fruits and vegetables had to travel from, with the most imported items coming from Mexico, Canada, China, and Costa Rica.

Fast Fact

Since so many fruits and vegetables in the produce aisle don't come with a label defining specific portion sizes, this will give you an idea of what a "serving" is equivalent to:

One cup refers to a common measuring cup (the kind used in recipes). In general, 1 cup of raw or cooked vegetables or 100 percent vegetable juice, or 2 cups of raw leafy greens can be considered as 1 cup from the vegetable group. One cup of fruit or 100 percent fruit juice, or ½ cup of dried fruit can be considered as 1 cup from the fruit group.

How to Shop for *Canned* Fruits and Vegetables

This type of packaging of fruits and vegetables has both advantages and disadvantages. Canned fruits and vegetables are often more cost effective, easier to stock up on, and have a long shelf life. Nutritionally speaking, canned fruits and vegetables are merely cooked, and their nutrient profile is similar to that of fresh. Some studies have shown that the fiber in canned fruits and vegetables may be easier to digest than that in fresh. Lycopene, a powerful antioxidant found in tomatoes, may even be more readily available to us in cooked or canned foods than fresh.

A disadvantage of canned vegetables is that the sodium content is higher than that of fresh. Check your Nutrition Facts Panel to see how much sodium you're getting per serving.

When to Can the Can

When purchasing any type of canned goods, watch out for dents or pockets of air in the cans. This can indicate bacterial growth, which could be harmful to your health.

What to Look for on the Label

Pay attention to these sections of your food label when shopping for canned fruits or vegetables:

Sodium content: As with many other canned goods, pay attention to the sodium content on your food label. Draining your fruits and vegetables is highly recommended. Rinsing canned vegetables can reduce sodium content by 20 to 40 percent. Otherwise, you might want to opt to buy the low-sodium (less than 140 mg or 5 percent of the Daily Value for sodium) or sodium-free-labeled cans when possible.

Sugar: Always look to see what type of liquid your canned fruit or vegetable is packed in (syrup, water, etc.). Usually this is written on the front of your can's label. Be careful, as these liquids can provide an additional source of calories as well as sugar. Many canned fruits will have a significant amount of added sugar. Remember, fruit is a natural source of sugar. The new NFP will differentiate between natural and added sugar. Look for statements on the label that say, "no added sugar" or "packed in its own juice" or "water packed." The best way to tell if added sugar is present is to look at the ingredient listing for words like high-fructose corn syrup and other names used for added sugar. Either buy the lighter options, or drain or rinse your fruits and vegetables after you open the can.

How to Shop for *Frozen* Fruits and Vegetables

Frozen fruits and vegetables are prepared by blanching and then freezing them. This process involves boiling water and dipping the fresh produce in it for a short amount of time (sometimes just mere seconds) and then freezing it. Most frozen produce is processed when it is ripe. According to the Food and Drug Administration, frozen fruits and vegetables provide the same type of nutrients as fresh fruits and vegetables with a minimal amount of processing. And with frozen produce, the price is usually better, too.

When purchasing frozen fruits and vegetables, follow the same principles as with fresh: Incorporate as many different colors as possible to make sure you're getting an array of important nutrients. Check the Nutrition Facts Panel and ingredient list for sugars, calories, and sodium, as mentioned earlier, especially when it comes to the packing medium. Fruits can be packed with unnecessary added sugars and frozen vegetables can include sauces and flavor packets high in sodium, fat, and calories.

What to Look for on the Label

COOL: This part of the label shows the country of origin for all imported goods, including frozen produce; it is required by the U.S. Customs Service. Although the front of the pack of frozen fruits and vegetables is supposed to mention "product of (country)" in a conspicuous spot, it is not always the case, and in some products, this information is missing altogether or difficult to read.

Flash frozen: This term refers to foods that have been frozen very quickly (usually within seconds) and is often sold in vacuum-sealed airtight packages. This process preserves flavor as well as vitamins and minerals.

How to Shop for *Dried* Fruits and Vegetables

Dried fruits are created through the removal of the product's water content. Dried fruit is chewy in texture and high in fiber, and in some cases other nutrients such as iron. You may also notice more freeze-dried products in your supermarket these days. These fruits and vegetables are produced in a process whereby moisture is removed from the frozen product using a very low temperature and a vacuum. Very little moisture remains in the product at the time of packaging, resulting in a product that weighs about 90 percent less than the original item, while the volume stays the same. This process concentrates the taste, natural color, and texture of fresh foods in their freeze-dried state. When rehydrated with water, the product will maintain the texture and shape of fresh product. Freeze-dried and dehydrated products are easy to store at home and their light weight makes them easy to travel with for quick, nutrient-packed snacks. Freeze-dried fruits and vegetables can be stored effectively for long periods of time and many do not contain additives or preservatives.

What to Look for on the Label

Calories: Dried fruits, although concentrated in nutrients, can also be concentrated in calories. Check the serving size as well as the calories. The key is to eat these treats in moderation.

Sugar: The sugars naturally found in fruit include fructose and glucose. With fruits that are naturally tart, such as cranberries, sugar may be added to enhance flavor. It's important to check the ingredient list to identify other sources of sugar.

Sulfites: Sulfites are often added to dried fruit to preserve them. If you are allergic to sulfites, it is imperative that you pay attention to the ingredient list on all packages of dried fruit. Thanks to FDA labeling regulations, sulfites are easier to identify on food labels: Look for sodium sulfite, sulfur dioxide, sodium and potassium bisulfite, and sodium and potassium metabisulfite on the ingredient list or the words, "contains sulfites" on the package.

Produce: Why you should be eating these powerhouses of nutrients

The following is a quick reference developed by the Kansas State University Agricultural Experiment Station and Cooperative Extension Service to help you identify good sources of the following important nutrients in the produce aisle:

Vitamin A: apricots, cantaloupe, honeydew, nectarines, plums, watermelon, broccoli, carrots, greens, winter squash, sweet potatoes, and tomatoes

Vitamin E: apples, apricots, nectarines, peaches, and greens

Vitamin C: apples, blackberries, cantaloupe, honeydew, nectarines, peaches, pears, plums, raspberries, strawberries, watermelon, asparagus, snap beans, broccoli, cabbage, cauliflower, greens, leafy lettuce, onions, bell peppers, summer squash, winter squash, sweet potatoes, and tomatoes

Thiamine: cantaloupe, honeydew, watermelon, and corn

Riboflavin: broccoli and sweet potatoes

Niacin: potatoes

Vitamin B_6: watermelon, potatoes, and sweet potatoes

Folate: asparagus, broccoli, cauliflower, corn, leafy lettuce, and greens

Calcium: broccoli and greens

Magnesium: broccoli

Iron: apricots

Copper: potatoes, sweet potatoes, and greens

Potassium: apricots, cantaloupe, honeydew, nectarines, peaches, pears, watermelon, asparagus, beans, cauliflower, corn, potatoes, winter squash, sweet potatoes, and tomatoes

Dietary fiber: apples, apricots, blackberries, nectarines, peaches, pears, raspberries, strawberries, snap beans, broccoli, cabbage, carrots, potatoes, winter squash, sweet potatoes, and tomatoes

---

Additive Alert: Be especially careful about these additives in fruits and vegetables

Artificial colors: Many foods are colored with combinations of synthetic dyes like Blue No. 2, Green No. 3, Red No. 40, and Yellow No. 5. Although the FDA banned Red No. 3 from many foods and cosmetics because of its link to thyroid tumors in rats, it's still being used. You'll find it in maraschino cherries. The concern is that synthetic dyes cause cancer. Yellow No. 5 must be listed on ingredient labels to prevent allergic reactions like hives, a runny or stuffy nose, or breathing difficulties in those people who are sensitive. Artificial colors have also been linked to hyperactivity in children.

Aspartame: Sold as NutraSweet or Equal, aspartame appears in diet fruit drinks and may cause dizziness, headaches, epileptic-like seizures, and menstrual problems in those that are sensitive and has been shown to increase the incidence of brain tumors, lymphomas, and leukemia in rats. Individuals who have phenylketonuria (PKU) are unable to tolerate products containing this artificial sweetener. An accumulation of phenylalanine in the blood of a baby with PKU can result in mental retardation. All packaged foods that contain aspartame carry warnings.

Butylated Hydroxyanisole (BHA): This chemical prevents oxidation and delays rancidity in foods that contain oil. Although it is potentially carcinogenic, it appears in hundreds of processed foods. The FDA currently considers BHA GRAS, or generally recognized as safe, although according to the EWG, the National Toxicology Program classifies BHA as a possible human carcinogen. Chips and preserved meats may contain BHA.

Monosodium Glutamate (MSG): For those who are sensitive, MSG can cause headaches, tightness in the chest, and a burning sensation in the forearms and the back of the neck, commonly known as "Chinese restaurant syndrome." If MSG is present, it must be labeled on the food package. Those who need to avoid MSG should avoid hydrolyzed vegetable protein (HVP), which may be listed on packages as "flavoring." MSG is commonly found in prepared vegetable dishes.

Chapter 10

Power-Packed Protein: Lean Meat, Poultry, Fish, Eggs, Beans/Legumes, Soy Products, and Nuts

Protein comes in all different shapes and sizes—from meat, to poultry, to fish, to tofu, and plantbased sources such as nuts, beans and legumes. Protein is an important part of your diet. It helps to repair and build muscle, boosts your immune system, and stabilizes your blood sugar levels—pretty important, wouldn't you say? You need a constant supply of protein from your diet in order to maintain the health of your entire body.

In general, we should get about 10 to 20 percent of our calories from protein, or 0.8 gram per kilogram of body weight per day. (Note: There are 2.2 pounds per kilogram, or kg, of body weight.) Some fad diets promote an excessive intake of protein, which could be unhealthy, unnecessary, and in some cases, even dangerous. When you take in more protein than your body needs, the excess doesn't go directly to your muscles, as many people believe—it actually can turn into fat. Certain groups, such as athletes or the elderly, may need more protein than others, and vegetarians need to be sure that they are consuming protein of good quality.

The buzz around plant-based eating is growing faster than the weeds in our backyards this summer—but you're not alone if you're not quite sure what it all means. Allow me to clarify: Plantbased eating doesn't mean placing your 16-ounce veal chop on a bed of greens, nor does it mean that you have to become a strict vegan or vegetarian. This style of eating basically means that meat (and other animal products) takes a step to the side while letting plants play the starring role on your dinner table.

A diet rich in vegetables and other produce has been shown to reduce risk for chronic diseases like heart disease, diabetes, and cancer. And, besides keeping people healthy, plant-based eating can also benefit our planet by decreasing global greenhouse gas emissions caused by food production practices, according to research published in _Nature._

I know what you're thinking: How can I possibly get enough protein in a meal without meat? It can be done! Combine a couple of plant-based protein sources into your meal and you can rack up more protein than you think. And considering the Institute of Medicine recommends a baseline of 56 grams of protein per day for men and 46 grams for women, you may not need to eat quite as much as you think. Of course, personal protein needs may vary depending on your goals, height, weight, and activity level, but many of us tend to go overboard on animal protein, eating steaks and burgers the size of our plates!

Fast Fact

Here's a quick protein primer:

Lean meat, like sirloin beef, top round veal, bison, and top loin pork, is a great source of iron, zinc, and B vitamins, although it may be one of the most expensive items on your shopping list. More research proves that you should limit your meat consumption to benefit your health and the environment, as well as your wallet, meat should be treated more like a side dish or incorporated into vegetable/grain dishes rather than treated as the main part of your meal.

Poultry is rich in B vitamins (especially B_6 and niacin) and minerals like iron, phosphorus, and selenium. Poultry is lower in saturated fat and cholesterol than red meat, that is, if you remove the skin. If you add a little skin to your bird, you'll be increasing the calories by 40 percent and more than doubling the saturated fat and total fat content.

Fishing for good health? Then fish is a great catch. Fish is lower in calories than meat or poultry and is rich in vitamins B_{12}, B_6, and D, iron, calcium, zinc, and more. It's full of omega-3 fatty acids, which multitask by helping your heart, improving brain function, reducing inflammation from arthritis, psoriasis, and asthma, and contributing to a long list of other health benefits.

Eggs are available year-round and provide high-quality, low-calorie, low-cost protein. They are rich in choline, and although they do contain cholesterol, they don't deserve the negative press they have gotten in the past. Dietary sources of cholesterol, as found in eggs, were believed to significantly contribute to blood cholesterol levels and the other laboratory values your doctor screens for when he or she checks your lipid profile through blood tests. It is now known that saturated fat, not dietary cholesterol, is the primary contributor to elevated blood cholesterol levels.

Soy products, such as tofu, are very good for you—they contains a potpourri of vitamins and minerals, including calcium, iron, potassium, phosphorus, and vitamin B, plus phytoestrogens (isoflavones) that have been shown to strengthen bones, stave off prostate cancer, reduce hot flashes, and support the heart.

Beans, often referred to as "the vegetable with more," uniquely provide a fat-free or low-fat, saturated fat–free and cholesterol-free source of protein. Beans can actually *lower* cholesterol and triglyceride levels.

Nuts provide an array of antioxidants and vitamins and minerals, like vitamin E, magnesium, selenium, magnesium, copper, phosphorus, potassium, and folate, as well as healthy monounsaturated fats. They are a proud member of the Protein Group of the *Dietary Guidelines for Americans*; 1 tablespoon of peanut butter or ½ ounce of nuts or seeds can be considered as a 1 ounce equivalent from the protein category.

Cheese is an excellent source of protein, calcium, vitamin D, and many other important nutrients. One cup of dairy is equivalent to 1 ½ ounces of natural cheese or 2 ounces of processed cheese.

Lean Meats

How to Shop for Meats

In order to minimize saturated fat intake, look for the leanest cuts of meat, and choose those that have the least amount of marbling. Usually those that include the words ***round*** or ***loin*** are lowest in fat content; they include:

- Eye of round
- Top round
- Bottom round
- Round tip
- Tenderloin
- Sirloin
- Center loin
- Top loin

When fresh meat is packaged, it sometimes has a purple tinge to it. This doesn't mean the meat is contaminated or dangerous to eat. Meat contains a color pigment called myoglobin that is purplish-red in color. When the meat is exposed to oxygen, the myoglobin undergoes a chemical reaction in which the pigment turns bright red. If you buy meat that has been vacuum-packaged, it hasn't been exposed to oxygen and thus will appear purple.

What to Look for on the Label

Principle Display Panel (PDP): Includes the name of the product, the net quantity of contents, the official inspection legend, the number of the official establishment, and in some cases a handling statement. Look for these three bits of information:

- **USDA Prime:** Very tender, very juicy, but the highest degree of marbling, and therefore the highest degree of fat.
- **USDA Choice:** This is the type of meat is easy to find in your local supermarket. It is slightly lower in marbling than USDA Prime, and is therefore lower in fat. It is still tender, juicy, and flavorful.
- **USDA Select:** This type of meat has the least amount of marbling. It is probably the best choice to select if you are looking for a low-fat option.

Information Panel: This part of the label will contain the manufacturer, the nutritional content of the meat, and in some cases, safe handling instructions, such as proper cooking temperatures and suggestions for safe storage. Storage instructions may include words like "keep refrigerated" or "keep frozen." Following storage instructions is crucial to help prevent food-borne illness. In fresh meat, you may have to refer to the back of a package to find the nutrition information.

Cured: Cured meats have been processed with a salt solution in order to improve flavor. Curing ingredients often include salt, spices, sodium phosphate, sodium nitrite, and sugars.

Cured (dry): These meats are not soaked in a solution but instead covered with salt and seasoning and left to dry for a longer period of time than wet-cured meats. Some meats that undergo this type of processing include prosciutto, country hams, and dried beef.

Cured (honey): Honey is added to the curing solution before the ham is cooked. While honey is a source of added sugars, the amount you actually get per slice of meat probably will be minimal.

Cured (wet): Wet-cured meats are soaked in a salt brine solution for several days. Meats that are processed this way include ham, sausage, pastrami, and corned beef.

Free-range, free-roaming meat or poultry: Although these animals must have access to the outdoors, no one is checking on them to see how much time they actually are spending outdoors.

Glazed: Deli meat that is coated by a glaze on the outside in order to give it a sweet flavor.

Grain-fed meat: The animals are fed a conventional diet of soybeans and corn.

Grass-fed meat: The livestock have access to fresh air, sunlight, and freedom to graze (access to pasture). It's important to note, however, that the food label doesn't tell you how long the cattle were in the pasture, and they *don't* have to be *exclusively* grass fed; these animals can also be given corn or soybeans. These animals *may or may not* be organic; if their feed is organic, they would be in compliance with government organic standards and therefore would be labeled accordingly.

Grass-finished meat: These animals are *exclusively* fed grass. They're "finished," or fattened, on grass, rather than grain, for the 90 to 160 days before slaughter.

Grass-fed and grass-finished animals also carry a lower carbon footprint (and are therefore better for the environment) because they emit less methane gases, as the grasses they consume are more digestible than grains. They also get sick less often and need fewer treatments with antibiotics. The meat from grass-fed/finished animals contains a slightly better nutrient profile, as they are lower in fat content and richer in vitamin E and conjugated linoleic acid (CLA), a fat that has many health benefits, as well as omega-3 fatty acids. (But if your diet is falling short on omega-3s, you may want to put fish on your plate instead of beef.)

But is the grass always greener? In terms of the environment, it takes far more water and energy to produce one meat-based meal than it does one grain-based meal. And even if a cow is fed grass, it doesn't necessarily qualify for the organic seal. Grass pastures can be maintained through chemical fertilizers and pesticides and farmers may use hormones and antibiotics, as there are no standards for grass-fed meat.

What's even more confusing is that cattle that are fed grain (and not grass) can qualify for the organic label provided they are raised and processed according to organic standards. Certified organic beef that has been grain fed may not have the nutritional benefits of grass-fed beef (as mentioned above).

Kosher meat (and poultry): The following animals are among those considered to be kosher: bison, cow, deer, goat, sheep, chicken, turkey, Cornish hen and goose. Meat and poultry require special preparation: animals must be slaughtered in a humane manner and with a special razorsharp, perfectly smooth blade, causing instantaneous death with no pain to the animal. After this process, a trained inspector checks the internal organs for any physiological abnormalities. It should be noted that in addition to fulfilling the requirements of Jewish law, this process ensures a standard of quality that exceeds that of the government. The meat or poultry is then soaked and salted to remove blood. "This is the reason they are often deemed better-tasting and the result is similar to the effect brining would have in the kitchen of a good chef," says Susie Fishbein, author of numerous cookbooks, including *Kosher By Design Lightens Up* (ArtScroll 2008), a project we collaborated on together. Many nonkosher consumers choose to buy meats and poultry bearing the kosher label, as aside from being tastier, kosher meats are considered to be cleaner and healthier. An important matter, however, is the sodium content. Meat and skin of kosher chicken can have four to six times as much sodium as nonkosher chicken because of the salt used in the process of Kashruth (koshering).

Kosher meat and poultry must be packed in tamperproof packaging with the kosher logo prominently displayed, and a metal tag bearing the kosher symbol is often clamped on the product to serve as an identifying seal of supervision until it reaches the consumer.

Extra-Lean: Meats that are labeled extra-lean contain less than 5 grams of fat, of which no more than 2 grams is saturated. These meats also contain less than 95 mg of cholesterol per 100 grams.

Lean: These meats usually contain less than 10 grams of fat, of which 4.5 grams (or less) is saturated. In addition, lean meat is required to have less than 95 mg of cholesterol per serving or per 100 grams (about 3 ounces).

Mechanically separated meat: A pastelike and batterlike meat product produced by forcing bones with attached edible meat through a sieve (or similar device) under high pressure to separate the bone from the edible meat tissue. Government regulations enacted in 2004 to protect consumers against bovine spongiform encephalopathy (mad cow disease) have prohibited mechanically separated beef for use as food for humans. However, mechanically separated pork is permitted; it must be labeled as such in the ingredient listing.

Fast Fact

A big BTW is that a label can say, "no hormones have been administered," but a label boasting "hormone-free" is false and illegal because all animals produce their own hormones.

Natural: The term "natural," as with all other products, does not mean organic. Producers that put the word "natural" on their meat and poultry labels do not have to undergo or adhere to the same specific guidelines that organic producers do. According to the Federal Register, livestock used for producing meat and meat products has to be raised entirely without growth hormones or antibiotics and is never fed animal by-products. The rule applies to all kinds of meat, including chicken, pork, beef, lamb, or goat.

No antibiotics: The term "no antibiotics added" may be used on labels for meat products if sufficient documentation is provided by the producer to the FDA demonstrating that the animals were raised without antibiotics.

No hormones: The term "no hormones administered" may be approved for use on the label of beef products if sufficient documentation is provided to the FDA by the producer showing no hormones have been used in raising the animals. Since hormones are not supposed to be used in raising hogs, the claim "no hormones added" cannot be used on the labels of pork unless it is followed by the statement "Federal regulations prohibit the use of hormones."

Organic meat and poultry: When it comes to organic meat, poultry, and fish, you might want to think of it as, "You are what *they* eat." The term also means that these products were not offspring of cloned animals. If you want to choose organic meat, look for the "certified organic" seal. To meet USDA standards, this meat will come only from animals fed 100 percent organic feed and given no hormones or antibiotics, and their meat was never irradiated.

Restructured meat: This term refers to several pieces of the meat bound together and shaped into one large piece of meat. Types of meat that can be restructured include beef and ham.

Sodium: When shopping for meats that aren't fresh, such as deli meats or sausages, pay close attention to the sodium and fat content on the nutrition label. When purchasing deli meats, be sure to read the front of the label, too. (Reminder: "low sodium" means 140 mg of sodium or less per serving.)

Smoke (artificial): A smokelike flavor is created by chemicals.

Smoke (natural): The meat is roasted or cured in the presence of natural wood smoke.

Smoke (natural flavor): This type of treatment doesn't actually involve smoking—smokelike flavoring is added during the curing process to develop the flavors.

Smoked: The meat is cooked in a smoke house using wood such as hickory, oak, Applewood, or mesquite.

Salty Meats—"Sometimes" Foods

Here are a few meats you should eat very rarely because of their nutritional profiles:

Ham: Contains about 3 grams of fat per 100 grams. Ham can be high in salt, and packaged ham is often made from off cuts of pork that are ground and reconstituted with water, starch, and additives and then pressed together. Buy the leanest ham (lowest in fat) possible with the least amount of visible white fat marbled through it. Fresh ham is leaner and lower in fat and salt than deli ham.

Bacon: If you are a bacon lover . . . save this food for your birthday! One strip provides 46 calories, of which 33 calories comes from fat, half of which is heart-harming saturated fat. This one strip also gives you 200 mg of sodium, as well as nitrites, which some food scientists believe to be cancer-causing.

Frankfurters: An average beef hot dog has 149 calories, of which 120 calories comes from fat. One dog supplies a whopping 513 mg of sodium. Maybe you should bring a sandwich to the game instead of getting that ballpark frank. You'll also find that that hot dog comes with a side of nitrites, so proceed with caution and make this a "sometimes" food, not a staple.

Poultry

How to Shop for Poultry

When shopping for poultry, it is important to keep in mind a few facts:

Dark or white meat: Dark meat has a higher concentration of myoglobin (a red pigment). Myoglobin is found in the muscles that are used more frequently, and is higher in fat, cholesterol, iron, and calories. Poultry parts considered to be dark meat include thighs and drumsticks.

Ground poultry: Ground chicken and ground turkey can be great substitutes for ground beef because they contain a smaller percentage of total fat, saturated fat, and cholesterol. When purchasing ground chicken or turkey, look at the percent lean and percent fat label on the front of the package. Try to choose the lowest values of fat.

What to Look for on the Label

Like red meat, poultry has its own grading system:

- **Grade A:** Uniform fat covered, have a good conformation, free of disjointed or broken bones, are free of pinfeathers, exposed flesh, and discolorations; and, in the case of whole carcasses, have no missing parts. If frozen, Grade A poultry products must be free of freezing defects such as dehydration or excess moisture. This grade is commonly found in your supermarket.

- **Grade B:** May have an occasional cut or tear in its skin, not as attractive or meaty in appearance as grade A.

Cage-free/free-roaming/free-range poultry: Most chicken grown for meat is kept indoors, but these hens are not kept in cages. Although they have access to the outdoors, as with cows, no one is keeping close tabs on them to know how much free-roaming time they actually have.

Chemical-free: The term is not allowed to be used on a label.

Fresh poultry: This refers to raw poultry that has never had an internal temperature below 26°F.

Frozen poultry: The temperature of raw, frozen poultry is 0°F or below.

Fryer-roaster turkey: Young, immature turkey usually less than sixteen weeks old of either sex.

Hen or tom turkey: This optional designation represents the sex of the bird (hen being female, and tom meaning male).

Mechanically separated poultry: Produced using the same process as described above in mechanically separated meat, and must be labeled accordingly.

Natural: A product containing no artificial ingredients or added color and is only minimally processed (in a way that does not appreciably alter the raw product) may be labeled natural. The label must elaborate upon the use of the term "natural" (such as "no added colorings").

No antibiotics: The term "no antibiotics added" may be used on labels for meat or poultry products if sufficient documentation is provided by the producer to the FDA demonstrating that the animals were raised without antibiotics.

No hormones: Since hormones are prohibited in for use in raising poultry, the claim "no hormones added" cannot be used on the labels of poultry unless it is followed by the statement "federal regulations prohibit the use of hormones."

Organic: The term "organic" is strictly defined by the USDA National Organic Program to include poultry raised with no antibiotics, fed 100 percent organic feed, and given access to outdoors.

Oven-prepared: The product is fully cooked and ready to eat.

Oven-ready: The product is ready to be cooked.

Young turkey: Turkeys that are less than eight months old (either sex).

Fast Fact

Stringent FDA and USDA regulations require chickens to be weaned from all antibiotics well before processing, but if you are concerned about antibiotic use in poultry, chose organic poultry. The use of hormones has been illegal in U.S. poultry production since 1952.

Fish

How to Shop for Fish

When you are buying fresh fish, always check to see that it is displayed and stored properly on ice (or refrigerated) and in clean, sanitized cases. Make sure you are purchasing your fish from a reputable source. Feel free to ask those working at your local supermarket about the freshness of the fish (ask how often it comes in) and where your fish comes from. The flesh should be firm, the eyes should be clear, and it should not have a "fishy" odor. If you are purchasing smoked fish, make sure that it is shiny and glossy. Remember that smoked fish can be high in sodium, so ask for lowersodium options when possible (such as Nova rather than belly lox).

Avoid buying cooked fish that is displayed right next to raw fish. This can indicate potential cross-contamination, which may pose a risk of food-borne illness.

Years ago consumption of low-fat fish, such as flounder and sole, and the avoidance of high-fat types was recommended by health professionals, but that was before spotlights were shown on the magical powers of eicosapentaenoic acid (EPA) and docosahexaenoic acid (DHA), better known as the omega-3 fatty acids.

What to Look for on the Label

Bones: Some cans of salmon are marked "skinless and boneless" on the label, but this is not necessarily a better choice: About 4 ounces of canned salmon including the bones is equivalent in calcium to a cup of milk. Check the bottom of the Nutrition Facts Panel to see the percent Daily Value for calcium to determine how much of your day's requirement of calcium this one food provides.

Dolphin-safe label: Schools of adult yellow-fin tuna swim beneath large groups of dolphins, which clued fishermen in to where to find a catch. Fishing vessels used to chase the dolphins until near death or death. As many as half a million dolphins died every year due to this process until the enactment of the U.S. Marine Mammal Protection Act (MMPA) in 1972. The "dolphin safe" label, which came about in the late 80s, promised consumers that their tuna had been caught without deliberately setting nets on dolphins. By 1994, the entire U.S. tuna fleet was dolphin-safe. The MMPA banned the importation into the United States of tuna caught by countries that didn't adhere to "dolphin safe" practices. To date "dolphin safe" standards continue to prohibit chasing or netting dolphins.

Farmed or wild: Farmed fish may be smaller (and therefore lower in mercury), less expensive, and more plentiful, and could even have more omega-3 fatty acids than some wild fish because they are continually fed and don't deplete their fatty-acid stores; however, farmed fish tend to have more fat, and PCBs are stored in fat. PCBs are environmental contaminants that were banned in 1979 because they were links to cancer and other health problems. Fish absorb PCBs from both the environment and their food. Wild fish, on the other hand, have lower concentrations of PBCs, but as mentioned above, and may be higher in mercury. Mercury is consumed by smaller fish and then these fish are eaten by larger, predatory fish. The older and larger the fish, the higher it's levels of mercury since it accumulates over time. Wild fish are harder to come by. For example, wild salmon season runs mid-April through the end of August; fresh wild fish is not always available. When it comes to a fish like salmon, canned is convenient (it's precooked) and more affordable than fresh, and you can enjoy it year-round. The label will tell you whether the salmon is wild or farmed.

So which is best? The bottom line is that the benefits of fish outweigh the potential negative risks, and the answer might be to try to have a variety of the types of fish you consume. In any event, avoid the fish highest in mercury content mentioned above. To swim on the safe side, remove the skin and visible fat.

Organic seafood: The USDA has never defined organic as applied to seafood, so it is an unregulated term. Some domestic and international seafood companies are raising their fish and seafood in controlled environments, free of antibiotics and chemicals and fed organic feed.

Packing liquid: It's important to know whether the fish you're purchasing is packed in oil or water. Oilpacked fish can have seven times the amount of fat as water-packed canned fish and double the calories. Unless you're holding the mayo, go for the water-packed version. Water-packed, however, doesn't mean that the fish is low in sodium; the amount is about the same for both.

Sodium: When purchasing canned fish, be sure to check the label for the sodium content. An average can of tuna contains about 500 mg sodium for 4 ounces. Canned anchovies can really ring the bell, clocking in at 734 mg for 5 anchovies. Look for low-sodium labels on canned fish.

Tuna types: "White" meat tuna is made of Albacore tuna. "White," in the case of tuna, does not represent something more clean and pure. In fact, "white" tuna has more mercury and is less safe to eat than "light" types. Canned "light" tuna can include any combination of various types of tuna, and it is also likely to be less expensive. The word "chunk" written on the label means that the tuna will appear in small pieces rather than the "solid" kind, which contains firmer, larger pieces.

> **Fast Fact**
>
> Fish highest in mercury include shark, swordfish, king mackerel, and tilefish. The bigger and older the fish, the more mercury it has a chance to accumulate. "White" canned tuna has more mercury and is less safe to eat than "light" types.

Eggs

How to Shop for Eggs

It used to be easy to buy eggs, but now it might take you longer to read an egg carton that a short novel.

Eggs are classified according to the USDA grading system and bear a label of AA, A, or B. This grading structure indicates quality parameters, including freshness, with AA representing a superior rating. Eggs are also labeled according to their size (weight), including jumbo, extra-large, large, medium and small. Medium eggs are defined as heavier than 1.75 ounces, large are heavier than 2 ounces, extra-large are heavier than 2.25 ounces, and jumbo are heavier than 2.5 ounces. The most common size, Large, is the size usually referred to in recipes.

Inspect eggs for breaks or cracks before purchasing them, and be careful when packing them in your cart and shopping bag on your trip home from the store. Store eggs in the refrigerator in their original covered carton with the pointed end facing downward so they don't absorb odors or lose moisture. (Don't keep them in the refrigerator door.) They will stay fresh for about one month.

> **Health Concerns**
>
> **Cholesterol:** If you prefer, there are many different types of egg substitutes are available, like cartons of egg whites. These products can be prepared in the same fashion as you would eggs, as most items are in liquid form. Powdered eggs and egg whites can also be found on supermarket shelves, and can easily be used when baking or can be used in place of fresh eggs when reconstituted with water.

What to Look for on the Label

Antibiotic-free: This term is unregulated and difficult to verify, but it suggests that hens that laid the eggs were not given antibiotics. Use of such drugs might encourage the growth of antibioticresistant bacteria, causing unknown illness in humans. Antibiotics used by humans, such as tetracyclines, are banned for use on laying hens.

Brown eggs: The color of the shell tells you nothing about the egg's nutritional profile, taste, or how the laying hen was raised: Brown eggs come from chickens with brown feathers and white eggs come from chickens with white feathers.

Cage-free, free-range/free-roaming: Although these hens are not confined to cages, thousands may crowd the barn or warehouse floor. They generally do not have access to the outdoors, and if they do have access, it doesn't necessarily mean they take advantage of that freedom. Beak cutting is permitted. There is no third-party auditing of this practice unless the eggs are also certified organic. These eggs may or may not be organic.

Certified humane, raised and handled: This term speaks to how the hens are treated but not what they are fed. The birds are uncaged, often inside barns or warehouses; they may be kept indoors at all times.

Fertile: These eggs are laid by hens regularly exposed to a rooster, and likely were not caged. Fertile eggs are no more nutritious than nonfertile eggs. They're also more expensive to produce and they don't stay fresh as long as nonfertile eggs.

Hormone-free: The FDA banned the use of hormones—most notably diethylstilbestrol, or DES— in poultry in 1959, after they not only caused tragic health problems in consumers but also failed to stimulate growth in chickens. As with other poultry products, "Hormone-free" is a not allowed to be used on labels unless it is followed by the statement "Federal regulations prohibit the use of hormones."

Natural: With most foods, "natural" is an unregulated term and does not designate a food as healthy in any particular way. When it comes to meat and poultry products, USDA defines "natural" as being free of artificial colors, flavors, sweeteners, preservatives and ingredients that do not occur naturally in the food. Unless the eggs have been pasteurized, eggs are natural. This term has no relevance to animal welfare.

Omega-3 enriched: Eggs that are higher in brain-boosting and heart-healthy omega-3s that come from hens that have been fed a diet rich in algae, ground flaxseeds, or fish oil. Although this is a nice addition, fish or walnuts are a better source of omega-3s.

Organic/certified organic: All organic eggs are certified by the USDA, and they generally cost more money. Organic eggs come from hens whose feed is free of pesticides, herbicides, fungicides, and commercial fertilizers, they have never been given antibiotics, and they are cage-free with access to the outdoors. Organic chicken feed contains no animal by-products.

Pastured/pasture-raised: Pastured hens range outdoors freely, and are given an organic diet (without hormones or nonorganic additives) and/or raised without antibiotics (drugs that are intended to prevent or treat animal illnesses). These hens are also able to eat grass, worms, bugs, fruit, and nuts in pasture. These eggs may have a slightly enhanced nutrient profile (more omega3s, more vitamins).

United Egg Producers certified: The overwhelming majority of the U.S. egg industry complies with this voluntary program, which basically ensures that hens are fed food and water. The UEP Certified program claims that hens also receive adequate space, proper lighting, and fresh air daily. What it doesn't tell you is whether their hens are confined in restrictive, barren battery cages and subject to cruel and inhumane factory farm practices.

Vegetarian/vegetarian diet: This label is supposed to tell you about whether the laying hen was on a vegetarian diet (no animal by-products), but chickens are omnivores and their diets may include insects and worms as a side dish to the vegetarian feed provided by the farmers.

Fast Fact

If you want to be eggs-tra careful about the eggs you're buying, choose organic eggs, which come from hens whose feed is free of pesticides, herbicides, fungicides, and commercial fertilizers, they have never been given antibiotics, and they are cage-free with access to the outdoors.

Beans/Legumes

How to Shop for Beans and Legumes

You can buy beans in either dried or canned form.

Canned: Make sure the can doesn't have dents and that it's not bulging; dents may indicate bacterial growth, which could lead to food-borne illness. Cans that are bulging in any way should be discarded, no matter what the expiration date says.

Dried: If you are buying dried beans, look for legumes of uniform size and those that are glossy and not wrinkled.

Dry or canned: The term "dry" on the label does not refer to how the beans are packaged or their state of hydration. "Dry beans" is the agricultural term for bean seeds that dry in their pods until

97

they are fully matured and harvested. So canned pinto beans and unhydrated pinto beans packaged in a bag are both dry beans. The only significant difference is that canned beans don't require any cooking ahead of time and are ready to add to any dish as soon as you open the can.

What to Look for on the Label

Sodium content: Recent studies have shown that draining and rinsing canned beans can reduce their sodium content by about 40 percent. It's a simple process that can make a big difference.

Sodium Labeling on Packages

Sodium-free: Less than 5 mg of sodium per serving

Very low sodium: Less than 35 mg of sodium per serving weighs less than or equal to 30 grams, it contains less than 35 mg of sodium per 50 grams of the food

Low-sodium: 140 mg or less of sodium per serving

Light in sodium: At least 50 percent less sodium per serving than the regular version of the same food with no sodium reduction

Lightly salted: At least 50 percent less sodium per serving than the regular version of the same food (If the food is not "low in sodium," the statement "not a low-sodium food" must appear on the same panel as the Nutrition Facts Panel.)

Reduced or less sodium: At least 25 percent less per serving than the regular version of the same food

Unsalted, without added salt, no salt added: No salt added during processing, and the regular version of the food is normally processed with salt. As with other canned foods, if the food is not "sodium-free," the statement "not a sodium-free food" or "not for control of sodium in the diet" must appear on the same panel as the Nutrition Facts Panel.

Type of packing liquid: Canned beans may be packed in sauce. Look closely at the product label to see what kind of sauce your beans are prepared with. If they are, for example, Red Beans in Sweet Sauce, you may be getting more sugar than you expected, so check the Nutrition Facts Panel, especially the ingredient list, for any additional sugar, fat, and sodium from the packing liquid.

Refried beans are often baked with lard, a saturated, unhealthy fat. Check the ingredients listing and try to avoid ingredients like lard or partially hydrogenated fats. Many companies are making fat-free refried beans that can be doctored up at home with your own seasonings and spices.

Fast Fact

You don't have to avoid canned bean because of their sodium content. Draining and rinsing canned beans can reduce their sodium content by about 40 percent while still providing a wealth of essential nutrients.

Soy Products

How to Shop for Soy Products

There are many different types of soy products, including:

Soybeans: As with any bean, be sure they are not wrinkled or shriveled; look for beans that are shiny and smooth.

Tempeh: Fermented soybeans pressed into a cake form; higher in protein than tofu.

Miso: Soybeans and grains ground into a paste that is used in soups and sauces.

Soy milk: Be sure you choose one that's calcium fortified.

Soy nuts: These contain more protein than most nuts.

Soy flour: This flour has twice the protein of wheat flour.

Tofu: I always picture tofu wearing a camouflage-colored uniform because it takes on the taste of the seasonings, spices, and flavors of the foods it is combined with. It's a great substitute for protein foods like meat, poultry, or cheese. About 4 ounces of tofu is equivalent in protein to 1 ounce of meat. Tofu comes in cakes with a soft, regular, or firm consistency; firm tofu is the highest in calcium content, which you can check in the percent Daily Value section of the Nutrition Facts Panel. It is generally packed in water to keep it moist, and it should be date-stamped. Vacuum-sealed tofu will last longer but may not taste as fresh. Once opened, tofu should be stored in fresh water (change daily) and eaten within a week.

What to Look for on the Label

MSG: Since tofu and other soy products are generally somewhat bland-tasting, they are often processed with flavor enhancers; be sure to check the ingredient list to see which enhancers you're getting. Monosodium glutamate (MSG), for example, is a chemical compound that is often added to foods (particularly in Asian cuisine) in order to augment flavor and palatability. It contains onethird the amount of sodium as table salt (13 percent versus 40 percent for table salt). For those who are sensitive to its effects, MSG may cause health symptoms such as headaches, flushing, sweating, numbness, and chest pain. The FDA requires that monosodium glutamate be listed on labels of foods containing MSG.

Organic: Look for the word "organic" to be sure that your soy product was grown without pesticides, as opposed to the word "natural" which does not meet the same assurance.

Sugar: Unsweetened soy milk contains around 4 grams of sugar per cup. Some flavored types are sweetened with added sugars, like dehydrated cane juice, so check the ingredients list.

Nuts

How to Shop for Nuts

The FDA tipped its hat to the benefits of nuts in 2003 by issuing a "qualified health claim" for peanuts and certain tree nuts—almonds, hazelnuts, pecans, some pine nuts, pistachios, and walnuts. The claim reads: "Eating a diet that includes one ounce of nuts daily can reduce your risk of heart disease." Look for the above types, and don't forget about cashews and macadamia nuts.

When shopping for nuts, keep in mind that because of their high oil content, nuts can easily become rancid. When out of the package, you should be able to smell this rancid odor, but taste is a more reliable gauge than smell. Chopped nuts are generally more prone to rancidity than whole nuts, so take this into consideration when buying and storing them. Some people keep nuts in the fridge to retain freshness, and nuts in their shells (called "unshelled") will keep for a year or so if refrigerated. Out of their shells, nuts can be stored in an airtight container for four or five months in the refrigerator and for up to a year in the freezer.

Nut and seed butters: Nut and seed butters are composed of crushed nuts, resulting in a product that spreads like butter. In spite of the name, these butters do not contain butter or the saturated fats that butter holds. Warm, toasted whole-grain bread with crunchy almond butter and raspberry jam makes me very happy! Nut butters are high in protein, fiber, and essential fatty acids and are a much healthier option than fats like butter or margarine that are void of nutrient value.

Some nuts are more highly processed than others. Try to purchase them as close to their natural form as possible, and preferably not salted or covered in honey, molasses, or any other sugary coating.

What to Look for on the Label

Added sodium and sugar: Most nut and seed spreads are about 95 to 100 calories per tablespoon. Try to buy nut butters that contain only ground nuts; check the label's sodium and sugar values to see what else is added to your jar. The fat that's taken out in reduced fat peanut butter is often replaced with sugar or some other sweetener. It's not worth the switch, and you'll be trading the rich, decadent flavor of the nut for sugar.

Dry-roasted: This term on the label doesn't mean the nut is dry or low in fat, as many people believe. Dry-roasted means that the nuts have been roasted without oil. An ounce of dry- roasted nuts contains approximately the same calories and fat as oil-roasted nuts. Even when purchasing dry-roasted nuts, it's important to read the label to be sure that no additional ingredients such as sugar, corn syrup, or preservatives have been added.

Serving size: Often nut labels will display small, unrealistic serving sizes on the Nutrition Facts Panel to show low, misleading fat and sodium levels. Also check the "serving size per container" section of the panel to determine how many people are supposed to be eating out of that package: Remember that the numbers listed reflect *only one* serving.

Trans fat: Check the ingredient list and try to avoid partially hydrogenated fat. Stick to nut butters that do not contain these harmful trans fats.

Additive Alert: Be especially careful about these additives in protein foods

Artificial colors: Many foods that contain colorants include a combination of synthetic dyes like Blue No. 2, Green No. 3, Red No. 40, and Yellow No. 5. Although the FDA banned Red No. 3 from many cosmetics and some foods because of its link to thyroid tumors in rats, it's still being used in maraschino cherries. The concern is that synthetic dyes may cause cancer. Yellow No. 5 must be listed on ingredient labels to alert people with allergies or sensitivities who could have reactions such as hives, a runny or stuffy nose, or breathing difficulties. Artificial colors have also been linked to hyperactivity in children. Such colors and dyes may be present in processed foods such as hot dogs, candy, and certain mac and cheese dinners, and frozen kid's meals.

Monosodium glutamate (MSG): For those who are sensitive, MSG can cause headaches, tightness in the chest, and a burning sensation in the forearms and the back of the neck, commonly known as "Chinese restaurant syndrome." If MSG is present, the food package must reflect it. Those who need to avoid MSG should avoid hydrolyzed vegetable protein (HVP), which may be listed on packages as "flavoring." MSG is commonly found in sausages, hot dogs, meat tenderizers, and gravies.

Nitrites/nitrates: Sodium nitrite and sodium nitrate have been used as preservatives, colorings, and flavorings in bacon, ham, hot dogs, luncheon meats, corned beef, smoked fish, and other processed meats. Although nitrate is not harmful, it is converted to harmful nitrite by bacteria in foods and in the body. In turn, nitrites can form cancer-causing compounds called nitrosamines. Nitrosamine formation can take place in the stomach or via frying foods at high temperatures.

Propyl gallate: This preservative is used to prevent rancidity in fats and oils and has been linked to cancer. It appears in meat products and chicken soup base.

Chapter 11

Utterly Delicious: The Dairy Aisle

Milk, yogurt, and cheese, when consumed in their fat-free or low-fat versions, contain a powerhouse of nutrients. Milk and other dairy products are not only for kids, and they provide approximately 70 percent of the calcium consumed in this country. If you don't consume enough calcium, your body extracts it from your bones, resulting in weak, frail bones, which can eventually lead to osteoporosis. Milk also provides a wealth of protein, riboflavin, vitamins A, D, and B_{12}, magnesium, phosphorus, and potassium. To top it off, dairy products are a good source of protein. One cup of skim milk has a little more protein than one ounce of chicken, one egg, or one-half cup of beans. To preserve your bones, consume the recommended three cups (about 1,000 mg worth of calcium) of milk, yogurt, or other dairy products each day. Unless you have a specific medical or personal reason why you'd avoid these foods, dairy products should appear regularly on your shopping list.

Milk

How to Shop for Milk

Try to purchase low fat options in your milk aisle.

Keep in mind that fat percentages are based on the weight of the fat within the milk—the percentages do not refer to the calories. Looking at the chart below, you can see that even though 2 percent might seem like a small number, when it comes to milk, it represents 35 percent of its calories. Below are the common milk products and their fat content:

Type of Milk	Calories from Fat
Heavy cream	92%
Light cream	90%
Half-and-half	79%
Whole or 4% milk fat	46%
2% milk fat	35%
1% milk fat	20%
Skim or nonfat	0%

Heavy cream: Heavy cream, also known as heavy whipping cream, has a fat content of between 36 and 40 percent. You'll find 50 calories in each tablespoon of heavy cream.

Light cream: Don't be fooled by the name— "light" cream is not light in calories or fat. Light cream is 20 percent butterfat, and at 30 calories per tablespoon, it'll make you heavier than halfandhalf! It's called "light" cream because it's lighter than heavy cream.

Half-and-half: A 50/50 mixture of whole milk and cream, most often used in coffee and tea. This milk product is higher in fat than whole milk, containing 20 calories per tablespoon, of which 15 come from fat. If you love cream in your coffee, try making it the exception rather than the rule, especially if you drink several cups of coffee during the day. This practice could save you hundreds of calories a week.

Nondairy creamer: These creamers are basically made of sugars and vegetable oils. The fat used is often partially hydrogenated oils loaded with the trans fats you should avoid. Other oils that may be used, if not trans fats, are coconut or palm kernel oil or soybean, cottonseed, or safflower oil. Sugars are composed of corn syrup, maltodextrin, and sugar. Some brands contain sodium caseinate to create a creamier look and feel, but may not be kosher or suitable for vegans. Vegan nondairy creamers are made with soy, coconut or almond.

Whole milk: According to the National Dairy Council, whole milk has about 3.25 percent fat. However, other sources give numbers as high as 3.7 percent fat. Regardless of the percentage, most of the fat in whole milk is saturated fat, the type of fat we should be avoiding or limiting in our diets. An analysis of one cup of whole milk by WIC discovered that out of 8 grams of fat present, 5 grams were saturated.

Whole milk, however, is beneficial for toddlers. Children under the age of two require a lot of calories because they are growing and developing at an extremely fast rate. Whole milk can help to provide adequate calories for this period of growth and development.

2 percent milk: This type of milk has 2 percent fat, as stated on the label. Once again, saturated fat makes up more than 50 percent of the fat present in 2 percent milk (3 grams out of 5 grams fat total). This type of milk is usually a good "transition" milk for those attempting to make the switch over from whole milk to skim or low-fat milks because it has more flavor than skim milk but less fat than whole milk. One cup of 2 percent milk provides 120 calories (45 derived from fat).

1 percent milk: This milk has 1 percent fat by weight. A comparison of caloric value per one cup of 1 percent milk to one cup of whole milk shows a 50-calorie difference (150 calories in whole milk, 100 in 1 percent). Considering that the average recommendation for milk (or the equivalent amount of dairy) is three cups each day, this would add up to a 150-calorie difference, which amounts to 1,000 extra calories a week.

However, some research now suggests that fat dairy may be more beneficial than previously thought. The fat in low-fat milk boosts satiation and satisfaction you get from drinking it. Remember to consider the fat in your milk as part of your overall diet, not on its own.

Skim (nonfat) milk: Skim milk is synonymous with nonfat milk, containing 0 percent fat. If you're trying to shed a few pounds, this is by far the healthiest option. Skim milk has approximately half the calories found in whole milk.

Skim (nonfat) milk—protein-fortified: This milk tastes richer and creamier than regular skim milk. The calories of this beverage are equivalent to that of 1 percent milk (100 calories per cup). Protein and calcium are added, providing an additional 3 grams of protein and 100 mg of calcium per cup (totaling 11grams of protein and 400 mg of calcium). Note, however, that proteinfortified milk also provides more sugar than most milk, at 16 grams per cup as opposed to the typical 12 grams per cup.

Flavored milk: Flavored milk is milk with added flavoring and sweetener. Chocolate is one of the most popular flavors, but other flavors such as strawberry and banana are also tasty options. Flavored milk provides calcium as well as many of the other nutrients found in plain milk, such as magnesium and potassium. However, it also could travel with a substantial amount of sugar and calories. Milk contains natural sugar from lactose (about 12 grams per cup), but it's the added sugars that can push these flavored milks over the top. A cup of flavored milk contains an average of 4 teaspoons of added sugar (about 16 grams) in addition to its natural sugar.

A Tasty Bone Boost

One of the questions I get asked frequently by moms is whether adding chocolate to milk has an effect on calcium absorption, as chocolate contains oxalic acid, a substance which diminishes calcium absorption. Not only doesn't it have an appreciable effect, but having chocolate milk as an option may encourage some people to drink more milk. What I would do, though (to limit sugar intake), is add a very small amount of chocolate syrup or powder to skim milk or combine chocolate milk with some plain milk. You'll still get the sweet flavor, but the sugar content will be lower.

Lactose-free milk: Lactose is the primary sugar present in milk. For those who are lactose intolerance, lactose-free milk is an excellent alternative, as it contains the same nutrient package as regular milk, including calcium and vitamin D. The significant difference is that the lactose in lactose-free milk has already been digested. In lactose-free milk products, the lactase enzyme is added to raw milk during processing. This enzyme breaks down the sugar into glucose and galactose, the two smaller sugars that make up lactose. You can find milk that is 100 percent lactose free in skim, 1%, 2%, and regular, whole milk versions.

Evaporated milk: Evaporated milk comes in whole and nonfat options. The higher-fat whole milk type contains almost twice the calories, coming in at a whopping 336 calories per cup. Try nonfat evaporated milk and save yourself 136 calories per cup.

Buttermilk: Despite its name, buttermilk is actually low in saturated fat (about 1 gram per cup). Buttermilk is simply milk with an acid added to it. The most common way of making buttermilk is to add bacteria, which creates lactic acid as a result of fermentation. The acid makes the milk taste a bit sour. One cup of buttermilk provides 100 calories and 2 grams of fat, similar to 1 percent milk.

If a recipe calls for buttermilk but you do not have any in your refrigerator, you can make your own buttermilk by adding 1 to 2 tablespoons of lemon juice OR white wine vinegar to one cup of milk.

Is Raw Milk Safe?

Currently raw milk primarily refers to milk that has not been pasteurized (heated to kill microbes.) Eight U.S. states prohibit sales of raw milk, whereas the remaining states either allow the retail or farm sales of raw milk. Federal law prohibits transporting it for sale across state lines.

The dangers of drinking unpasteurized milk are plenty; food-borne illness can occur from harmful bacteria that are normally killed by pasteurization. Regardless of the health benefits, certain populations should be especially careful when purchasing unpasteurized milk. These include the elderly, the young, and those with compromised immune systems; pregnant women should avoid raw milk altogether.

What to Look for on the Label

Antibiotics: According to the USDA, all milk must be tested to make sure that any antibiotics that were used to treat the cows are not present in the milk. The FDA's 2007 National Milk Drug Residue Database Annual Report showed that out of the more than 3.3 million milk tankers that were tested on a mandatory basis at processing plants, only 0.032 percent (less than one in every three thousand) were positive for any animal drug residues, including antibiotics. When a tanker was found to be positive, the milk was disposed of, never reaching the consumer. Antibiotics are not administered to milking cows on a routine basis; they are only used to treat sick cows.

Fat: Full-fat dairy products contain saturated fat and cholesterol, so choose low- or no-fat (skim) items. Most people don't realize that you can slash the fat and calories of dairy and still retain a wealth of nutrients, including protein, calcium, and magnesium, just to name a few. In some cases, the nutrient content in skim products surpasses the profile of full-fat varieties, since some skim milks contain additional protein solids and calcium.

Homogenized: Homogenization is a process that distributes milk's fat molecules throughout the product. This creates an emulsion that prevents the cream from separating out from the rest of milk. Nonhomogenized milk that *has* been pasteurized poses no public health threat.

Hormones: Hormones *are* present in milk because all cows have a natural protein hormone (bST) that helps them produce milk, without ever adding any. Some dairy farmers choose to supplement their cows' rBST (also known as rBGH) to boost milk production. Although the FDA concluded that beef and dairy products derived from rBST-supplemented cows are safe for human consumption, some consumer and environmental groups fear that this hormone may have a negative effect on humans (possible cancer causing) and cows (causing udder inflammation, or mastitis.) A 2008 study in *Journal of the American Dietetic Association, however,* analyzed the composition of organic milk, milk labeled "rBST-free," and whole milk, and found that the label claims were not related to any meaningful differences in milk composition.

Organic: When shoppers are buying organic milk, their impression is that it is hormone-free, pesticide-free, and antibiotic-free, but no milk is truly "hormone-free," because cows naturally have hormones without adding any. Both organic and conventional milk generally have low pesticide levels, and if antibiotics are found in milk, the milk is then destroyed. So what should your decision be about buying organic milk? Even health professionals are mixed about that choice. The bottom line is that if you enjoy milk and all the benefits it provides, choose skim or low-fat milk, and if you have concerns about the use of antibiotics, hormones, and pesticides, organic skim or low-fat milk is a good option for you.

In addition to complying with the requirements of conventional dairy producers, such as providing them with comfortable living conditions, nutritious diets, and good medical care, organic dairy foods must also meet the requirements of the USDA's National Organic Program. This includes using only organic fertilizers and pesticides and not using any antibiotics or growth hormones like rbST. Dairy foods can be labeled "USDA Organic" only if all the additional criteria are met.

Milk and cheese from grass-fed cows has been found to have four times the amount of conjugated linoleic acid (CLA) than conventional milk and cheese. CLA is a naturally occurring type of fat; studies have shown that it may help regulate glucose metabolism, decrease cholesterol levels, boost the immune system, enhance bone formation, and reduce the incidence of certain cancers. Research has also shown that organic milk contains up to 70 to 240 percent more omega3 fatty acids than conventional milk, as well as a higher content of vitamin E, beta-carotene, and other important antioxidants.

Pasteurized: Pasteurization is a process of eliminating harmful pathogens in milk. This is done by exposing the milk to high heat for a specific period of time. Because this process involves heat treatment, in addition to destroying harmful bacteria, some beneficial bacteria are destroyed as well. The benefits of this process, which keeps milk safe, outweigh any negatives.

Percent Daily Value: Notice how milk has impressive numbers in the % DV section of your food label, including one-third of your day's calcium, as well as vitamins A and D and several B vitamins.

Pesticides: Since pesticides are found in the water and soil, extremely low levels of pesticides can be found in all foods—both conventional and organic. Thorough FDA and USDA testing has shown that milk ranks among the lowest of all agriculture products in detectable residues. Pesticides are never added to milk or milk products; thus the Federal Trade Commission has deemed manufacturers' "no pesticide" claims to be misleading.

Protein: One cup of milk provides about 8 to 11 grams of protein, the same amount that's in almost 1 1/2 ounces of meat or chicken. Some skim milk is fortified with protein to enhance taste and mouthfeel.

Trans fat in nondairy creamers: The fat in nondairy creamers may be composed of harmful saturated and trans fats. Many labels of nondairy creamers have improved the serving size to become more realistic. Most labels show 15-20 calories and almost 1 gram of saturated fat per serving, with the serving size of 1 tablespoon. After several cups of coffee including this whitener each day or the addition of 1 cup of nondairy creamer in place of milk in a recipe, you could be loading up on more fat than you realized.

Milk Alternatives

Milk alternatives provide benefits to people who are severely lactose intolerant, vegans, or just don't enjoy milk and other dairy products.

Almond milk: Almond milk may not have as many nutrients as the heart-healthy nut it is derived from, but it is fortified with calcium and vitamin D. Almond milk is also an excellent source of vitamin E and is a good source of vitamin A. Almond milk generally contains around 1 gram of protein for 8 ounces, as compared with 7 grams of protein in soy milk and 8 to 11 grams in skim milk. Some brands of almond milk contain sweeteners, so check labels carefully if you're looking to cut back on sugar. Considering that most of us get more than enough protein in our diets, almond milk can be a delicious alternative to those who focus solely on plant protein, those who have certain allergies or intolerances or those who simply enjoy its nutty flavor.

Soy milk: Soy milk is made from soybeans that have been ground up, soaked in water, and then strained. This liquid is high in protein, as it is made from a bean. Since soy milk is lower in calcium and vitamin D than cow's milk, it's best to purchase a brand that is fortified with these nutrients. Check the front of the package where calcium and vitamin D should be mentioned, and you can look at the percent Daily Value on the Nutrition Facts Panel (NFP) to see just how much you're getting. Some brands of almond milk contain sweeteners, so check labels carefully if you're looking to cut back on sugar.

Rice milk: Rice milk is made with rice, some type of sweetener, and rice syrup. Because the origin of this milk alternative is a grain, rice milk contains double the carbohydrate content of cow's milk (24.8 grams versus 12 grams per cup). This beverage can also be fortified with calcium and vitamin D but falls short in other important nutrients present in cow's milk or soy milk, such as protein.

Cashew milk: Cashew milk does not contain nearly as many nutrients as other milk alternatives, but it is the lowest calorie option with only 25 calories per cup. Cashew milk is typically fortified with vitamins A, D and E, as well as calcium, but contains less than 1 gram of protein per serving.

Coconut milk: Coconut milk is another popular alternative for individuals who are allergic to dairy, almonds and soy. Coconut milk contains more fat than almond milk, most of which is saturated fat. Coconut milk typically contains about 4.5 grams of fat, of which 4 grams is saturated fat with no protein. However, there are some nutritious benefits to coconut milk as it is usually fortified with calcium, vitamins A, D and B12 and calcium. Some brands of almond milk contain sweeteners, so check labels carefully if you're looking to cut back on sugar.

Be sure to opt for unsweetened varieties of these milk alternatives to avoid excess added sugar consumption.

Yogurt

The yogurt aisle in the supermarket seems to be growing faster than the bacterial cultures nestled within! Yogurt is one of those foods that has a health halo around it; people just automatically assume it's good for you. In many cases, yogurt's "active live cultures" and friendly bacteria can help settle your stomach, relieve constipation, and soothe several other gastrointestinal ailments. Yogurt is also rich in calcium, phosphorus, and other vitamins and minerals.

Yogurt is made by adding bacteria to milk; the bacteria release an acid that causes the milk to ferment. The fermentation process helps to digest some of the lactose, making digestion easier. For this reason, yogurt sometimes can be tolerated by people who are lactose intolerant.

How to Shop for Yogurt

Not all yogurts are alike. Right beside yogurts that are filled with active cultures, calcium, and a variety of other rich nutrients, your dairy case will also hold flavored, highly sweetened yogurts that are like candy in a container instead of a valuable dose of dairy.

Low-fat yogurt: These products are made with low-fat milk that ranges from 0.5 to 2 percent fat. One cup has about 150 calories, 5 grams of fat, and 400 to 450 mg of calcium.

Nonfat yogurt: This yogurt is made from nonfat (skim) milk that is less than 0.5 percent fat. One cup has about 80 to 130 calories (depending on whether artificial sweeteners are used), 0.4 gram of fat, and 400 to 450 mg of calcium. Remember that Food and Drug Administration regulations allow for up to 0.5 gram of fat for a product to be labeled as "nonfat."

Greek yogurt: This type is usually thicker in texture because it has been strained to remove the whey. It contains between double and triple the amount of protein found in most other yogurts and is generally lower in sugar as well as carbohydrates, making it healthier and easier to digest. Flavored types may contain more sugar than you'd like, so be sure to check the new food labels when they come out so that you'll be able to tell the difference between the natural sugar within yogurt (lactose from milk and sugar from fruit) and the added sugar the manufacturer put in their product.

You might also notice that there's a surge in popularity of full-fat Greek yogurt in stores. If I have patients that say they don't like Greek yogurt, I might suggest that they try a full-fat type; it's creamier, tastier and just as rich in benefits as the lower fat types. It's just higher in calories and fat which, in some cases, is worth the calories when looking at the total nutrition profile (benefits) of the food. I've often seen someone start out will full-fat Greek yogurt and then trim down to fatreduced versions once they develop a liking for this product.

Drinkable yogurt: The American lifestyle is certainly one filled with many "grab-and-run" meals and snacks. Drinkable yogurts have been created specifically to fit in with our fast-paced lives, but they come with both benefits and drawbacks. On one hand, they provide a healthier alternative to high-fat snacks such as chips, cookies, and candy, but as with any yogurt, it is important to pay attention to the sugar content and the list of ingredients. Many drinkable yogurts intended for kids are filled with added sugars and fruit-flavored drinkable yogurts often contain very little actual fruit. For adults, a more mindful experience (eating slowly with a spoon instead of drinking it), may help to cut calories through the appreciation of yogurt's creamy texture.

Kefir: This fermented milk beverage was commonly found in Slavic diets and is now found in most stores. Like American-style yogurt, kefir is made by fermenting milk. Kefir is different in texture from yogurt, because making it involves working with kefir "grains," which are a mixture of bacteria, yeast, and milk proteins. Kefir provides many of the same nutrients found in other dairy products, including protein, calcium, phosphorus, magnesium, and B vitamins and vitamin D. Kefir, like Greek yogurt, often contains less sugar than American-style yogurt, and can be incorporated in your meals in a variety of ways. Although yogurt often can be digested by lactoseintolerant people, kefir is often even easier to digest. As with American-style yogurts, kefir can come in many varieties—flavored, nonfat, low-fat, and full-fat, so read the label for the percentage of fat and sugar. In addition, you may want to take note of what type of milk was used to make the kefir; kefir can be made with cow's or goat's milk, and there are soy-based versions available as well.

What to Look for on the Label

Additional ingredients: Some yogurts come with additional ingredients, such as granola or candy. Yogurt add-ins can be delicious and wholesome, but manufacturers often couple yogurt with foods that are not the healthiest options available. Be sure to read the Nutrition Facts Panel for the sugar, fat, and calorie content. If you enjoy the addition of a little crunch, skip the high-fat, highsugar granola that comes with some types of yogurt and add some of your own high-fiber, lowsugar cereal. In addition to saving calories, this option will save you money, too.

Fat content: Yogurt can be made with a range of fat content, depending upon the starting milk product. Check the label to see what type of milk was used: whole milk, 2 percent, 1 percent, or skim.

Ingredient label: Yogurt ingredient lists can range from very simple to incredibly long and complex. Try to choose yogurt with about five ingredients or fewer to ensure that the yogurt has undergone minimal processing, and avoid yogurt containing chemical additives.

Live cultures: When purchasing yogurt, always look at the label to see if your choice includes live cultures. This means it contains probiotics, live microorganisms that are beneficial in helping with digestion of food and regulation of the GI tract. Probiotics may also aid in preventing diarrhea, reducing inflammation in the GI tract, and boosting your immune system. Yogurt that contains live cultures may be easier to handle for lactose-intolerant people, as the bacteria it contains can help digest lactose.

Probiotics can also be sold as dietary supplements; they are not regulated by the FDA, but because probiotics are already part of our digestive tract naturally, they are considered to be safe.

The cultures that are often used include *Lactobacillus* and *Bifidobacteria.* These microorganisms colonize the intestinal tract and help to increase immunity and fight disease. They do so by adhering to the walls of the gastrointestinal tract, thereby preventing other, harmful bacteria from colonizing in your body. Ingesting probiotics can help to prevent various forms of diarrhea, as well as prevent the colonization of *H. pylori*, a bacteria responsible for causing ulcers and gastritis.

Sugar content: Although yogurt has plenty of health benefits, it's also often filled with added sugars and calories. Always be sure to check the Nutrition Facts Panel on your food label to see how many grams of sugar your yogurt contains and the ingredient list to see what type of sugar is added. Yogurt with whole "fruit on the bottom" will likely have more sugar because the fruit provides natural sugars. Natural sugar is better than high-fructose corn syrup and other sugars, but the best option is to add your own fruit to plain yogurt when possible. Always opt for the lowest sugar option. Plain yogurt may contain anywhere from 8 to 12 grams of sugar, from the lactose contained in milk.

Fast Fact

Believe it or not, even frozen yogurt contains live cultures. The freezing process causes the cultures to go into a dormant state, and when eaten and returned to a warm temperature within the body, they again become active and can provide all the benefits found in nonfrozen yogurt. Quality frozen yogurt will have a National Yogurt Association Live and Active Cultures (LAC) seal.

Yo!

Remember to check the calcium content of your yogurt. Unlike milk, whether skim or whole, where the amount of calcium is generally the same per serving, the calcium in yogurt can fluctuate dramatically: the same 8-ounce container can vary from 20 to 45 percent of the Daily Value.

Cheese

Cheese is a nutrient-rich food filled with vitamins and minerals and is also rich in protein. To be more specific, ounce for ounce, cheese measures up in protein content to meat, chicken, or fish. One and a half ounces of cheese has about the same amount of calcium as a cup of milk. For those who are lactose intolerant, cheese may be a safer option; because of the processing that most cheeses undergo, it is often easier to digest and therefore a good source of calcium for those who do not drink milk.

How to Shop for Cheese

Although cheese has many nutritional benefits, consumers must be careful to pay attention to the fat content listed on the label. Cheese is often classified according to its firmness (soft, semisoft, semihard, and hard), but this type of categorization is not exact. Generally, the softer the cheese, the higher the fat content, though this does not apply to cottage cheese, which usually is low in fat and calories. Even full-fat cottage cheese, which contains 4 percent milk fat, is relatively low in fat, though I recommend that you purchase low-fat (1 or 2 percent). Brie, cheddar, and Muenster cheese are among the highest in saturated fat content.

In terms of quality, before you buy, make sure that a cheese that is meant to be soft isn't hard (this indicates it is not fresh), and make sure that it isn't moldy (unless, like blue cheese, it is meant to be).

What to Look for on the Label

Aged cheese: Aged cheeses (aged nine months or longer) have been cured for longer than six months and generally have a more pronounced, fuller, and sometimes sharper flavor than mediumaged (aged four to five months) or current cheeses (see below).

Current (young): A mild-flavored cheese that typically is semifirm, firm, or hard in texture and has been cured for from two weeks to thirty days.

Fat content: Always look for the grams of fat or the percent of fat in the milk used (cheese is made from whole milk, 2 percent, 1 percent, or skim). Pay close attention to serving size as well. One ounce of cheddar cheese, for example, has 114 calories, of which almost 85 calories comes from fat. In addition, 54 of these 85 calories is artery-clogging saturated fat. There are low-fat cheddars on the market that cut the fat content in half, so check the Nutrition Facts Panels to be sure to choose the cheese that's best for you.

Fat-free cheeses, although lowest in calories and fat content, sometimes are rubbery in texture and they may not melt well. Your compromise may be to purchase cheeses that are *low* in fat (2 to 5 grams of fat per ounce) rather than fat-free.

Natural cheese versus processed cheese: Natural cheese is made from milk that has been allowed to thicken; a couple of common types are cheddar and mozzarella. Processed cheese is a blend of cheeses that have been treated with gelatin thickeners, emulsifying agents, preservatives, salt, and food coloring and have a smooth texture. They have also been pasteurized to lengthen their shelf life. Yellow American cheese is a type of processed cheese. U.S. government standards dictate that processed cheeses must contain at least 51 percent cheese. The remainder is made up of water, whole milk, skim milk, buttermilk, powdered milk, or whey.

Smoked cheese: Cheese that has been smoked in a process similar to smoking meat, including the addition of liquid smoke to the brine or smoking over wood chips.

Sodium: Some cheeses, particularly those low in fat, can be high in sodium. As a reminder when looking at cheese labels, the criteria for sodium labeling is as follows:
- Sodium-free (less than 5 mg sodium per serving),
- Very-low-sodium (35 mg or less per serving), or
- Low-sodium (140 mg or less per serving)

Spreads: Spreads come in a variety of flavors. They are usually loaded with sodium and without the nutrient value of natural cheese. If you add some spread to salty crackers, you may end up with your full day's sodium requirement in one quick snack.

As with natural cheese, the fat content of cheese spreads varies greatly, so be sure to pay attention to the calories from fat and the type of fat that's listed on the Nutrition Facts Panel. There are products available that are reduced in fat and sodium, and some that are even fat-free, but you might find that as the fat content decreases, the sodium content increases, so remember to take your particular health concerns into consideration when making your purchase.

> **Spread the News: Skip the Spreads:**
> Here's a quick comparison chart to help you make a wise shopping decision:

111

	Calories	Protein	Calcium	Sodium
Natural cheese 1 ounce	72	6.9 grams	183 mg	132 mg
Processed cheese 1 ounce	106	6.3 grams	175 mg	405 mg
Cheese spread 1 ounce	91	4 grams	118 mg	541 mg

Cream Cheese:
cream cheese

Cheese (1 ounce)	Cream cheese (1 tablespoon) I don't	think
Protein	7 grams	1 gram
Calcium	150–190 mg	12 mgs
Potassium	47–75 mg	17 mg
Fat	0–8 grams	0–10 grams

correctly reflects its name; "cream fat" would be more accurate. Cheese is a good source of calcium, protein, and an assortment of other important vitamins and minerals, but this is not what cream cheese is about. The following chart gives a comparison of the typical nutritional value of regular cheese and cream cheese.

Cream Cheese or Cream Fat?

Chapter 12

Going with the Grain: Breads, Cereals, and Starches

Whole Grains

Grains are our best source of energy, fiber, and a host of vitamins and minerals that no other group can provide. But this isn't a license to gorge—you'll need to focus on nutrient-rich whole grains and portions to make the most of the benefits of grains. You have a lot to gain (and I don't mean weight) by adding whole grains to your diet.

There is a lot of room for the grain group on the USDA MyPlate. We need about 6 servings of grains a day (with adjustments depending on particular requirements), of which at least half come from whole grains.

1 serving of bread/whole grains is equivalent to:
Whole-grain cereal = 1/2 cup cooked or 1 ounce of ready-to-eat
Whole-grain bread = 1 slice or 1 ounce
Whole-grain tortillas, muffins, waffles, pancakes = 1 small Popcorn = 2 cups
Whole-grain crackers = 5 to 7 small crackers or 1 ounce
Whole-grain bagel, pita bread = Half or 1 ounce Brown rice, whole grain pasta = 1/2 cup cooked

These days, we see and hear a lot about whole grains, but most people don't really know what they are. A grain is essentially a seed of a plant. It can be milled and refined into familiar foods such as pasta, rice, and bread. A whole grain is the entire seed; it consists of three main components:

the bran, the endosperm, and the germ.

Bran (about 15 percent of the grain): This is the outside of the grain. It is a wonderful source of fiber, vitamins, and phytochemicals (compounds in plants believed to reduce the risks of many diseases).

Endosperm (about 83 percent of the grain): The endosperm is mostly a source of carbohydrates, some protein, and a small amount of B vitamins. When you purchase a refined grain (like white bread), you are getting the endosperm of the seed; the germ and bran portions were removed during milling, the nutrient content was reduced by 25 to 90 percent, and then, in many products, some of the nutrients were put back in processing, or enriched.

Germ (About 2 percent of the grain): The germ of a grain contains a variety of essential vitamins and minerals as well as healthy, unsaturated fats. The presence of fats in the germ makes whole grains (and especially wheat germ) more prone to spoilage than refined grains, so it's best to refrigerate these products to prevent rancidity. The germ is a rich source of vitamin E, a potent antioxidant, as well as an abundance of B vitamins.

How to Shop for Grains

Don't be fooled by products that are brown in color. Often consumers confuse the color of a food for its whole grain value. The truth is that some brown-colored products (like bread and crackers, for example) have molasses added but aren't whole grain. Buying "dark" bread is not the same thing as buying whole grain bread. That's where the Nutrition Facts Panel and ingredient list come in handy.

Look for the following whole grains in your grocery aisle:
Amaranth
Brown rice
Buckwheat or kasha, buckwheat groats
Corn or cornmeal (yellow and white)
Cracked wheat (also called bulgur)
Millet Popcorn
Quinoa
Rolled oats (old-fashioned, quick, or instant)
Rye
Spelt
Teff
Triticale
Whole barley
Whole oats
Whole wheat pasta
Wild rice

Note: If you have celiac disease, you can still enjoy the whole-grain goodness of amaranth, brown rice, wild rice, buckwheat, cornmeal, millet, quinoa, and teff.

Fast Fact

Attention all carb lovers: Carbs are back. Complex carbs are a great source of energy and fiber, and they can boost your mood. But carb calories can add up: an average-size bagel (6 ounces) can be equivalent to 6 slices of bread. (That's almost 500 calories without the schmear!)

What to Look for on the Label

The FDA has specific regulations for what is considered whole grain, and which foods may be labeled as such. The FDA's definition of whole grain is: "*grains that consist of the intact, ground, cracked or flaked caryopsis, whose principal anatomical components—the starchy endosperm, germ and bran—are present in the same relative proportions as they exist in the intact caryopsis.*" Sounds pretty dry, doesn't it? This simply means that all three components of the whole grain need to be present for a whole grain to be classified as such.

Because consumers today are becoming increasingly health conscious, producers of grain products (both healthy and unhealthy) are doing all they can to advertise the whole-grain content of their products. Here are the symbol and claims you may see on food labels:

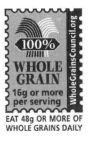

Figure 14. Whole Grain Stamp

Whole grain stamp: The whole grain stamp is an initiative of the <u>Whole Grains Council</u>. This stamp can be found on food products like bread, pasta, rice, and cookies. Every stamped product must contain at least half a serving (8 grams) of whole grains. Since it is recommended that an average adult eat at least three servings of whole grains every day, eating six products with this whole grain stamp will ensure that you are getting your full day's serving of whole grains. In accordance with the Whole Grain Stamp Program (Phase II), all whole grain–stamped labels must include the whole-grain content on the label. However, some products still use old labels; in this case, you'll see statements like:

Excellent source/100%: 16 grams or more of whole grains (remember, 16 grams is considered one serving).

Good source: 8 grams or more of whole grains. Remember, this is half a serving. So technically, *every* product with the whole grain stamp is a good source of whole grains.

The Whole Truth

It's important to remember that even if a product has the "whole grain stamp" it isn't necessarily a healthy food. The product's 8 grams of whole grain, although beneficial, can be offset by high levels of sugar, fat, and sodium. A tasty 8-ounce whole-grain muffin can set you back by 600 calories, providing almost a half day's worth of calories. Read the ingredient label to see *everything* you're getting.

Bran: This refers to the bran (outer) portion of the grain. Products containing bran (oat bran or wheat bran) in their ingredient list are often very high in fiber but may *not* actually be whole grains. Something very important to remember about high-fiber foods is that you may need to introduce them into your diet slowly and gradually to prevent uncomfortable reactions like gas, bloating, or gastrointestinal discomfort. You can minimize these side effects by increasing your fluid intake, particularly water.

Durum wheat: Consumers often confuse durum wheat for whole wheat. Durum wheat is a type of flour that is extremely high in protein and is used to make pasta (semolina is durum wheat). Durum wheat has had its bran and germ removed and therefore is not a whole grain.

Fiber: It's important to consume fiber on a daily basis, and, as mentioned earlier, whole grains contain more fiber than refined grains because of the bran. But this part may be a little tricky—not all high-fiber foods are whole-grain foods. You may wonder why a bran cereal that contains 16 grams of fiber per serving is *not* a whole grain—that's because bran is the outside *part* of a grain; it's not a *whole* grain. To make sure something is truly whole grain, check the ingredient listing.

Flour (enriched): Be careful! Enriched flour and fortified flour are often confused for each other. Enriched flour has had all of the vitamins and minerals that were originally present in the grain stripped away and then replaced. Usually these vitamins and minerals are lost during the food processing procedure.

Flour (fortified): This flour has had *new* vitamins and minerals placed into it, meaning those that weren't naturally present in the grain prior to processing.

There are pros and cons when it comes to fortifying foods. Fortification can be beneficial because it can help to prevent serious public health problems. For example, fortification of iodine in salt has helped prevent thyroid problems and goiter. Fortification of grains and flour with folic acid has prevented neural tube defects in children. Fortification of dairy products and orange juice with vitamin D has provided a good source of the vitamin that is not naturally present in many foods.

Manufacturers have begun to fortify all kinds of foods—white pasta is now fortified with fiber and protein, yogurt is fortified with fiber, and water is fortified with vitamins and minerals. Although fortified foods have their place on supermarket shelves, people often give such food health halos and mistake fortified but unhealthy options for healthier, fresh food sources. In addition, just like with any vitamin and or supplement, eating too much of a fortified food can cause vitamin or mineral overload and be dangerous to your health.

Flour (refined): This type of flour consists of mainly the endosperm of the grain (not the bran or germ). Many vitamins, minerals, and phytochemicals are lost throughout the refining process. Refined flour can raise blood sugar more readily than whole-grain flour and doesn't make us feel as full.

Ingredients: Ingredients are listed in order from highest concentration by weight in the product to lowest.

When purchasing grains, look for these words to appear first in your ingredients label:

> **Brown rice**: The FDA has recently allowed brown rice to carry a "whole grains logo." In the past, this wasn't the case because its fiber content was too low. However, rice is a staple food in many cultures and is consumed throughout the world; substituting brown rice for white rice is a great way to increase whole grain intake. **Side note:** Brown rice can be rinsed prior to cooking, while white

rice should *not* be rinsed. White rice is often enriched with vitamins and minerals, which would be lost in the water if the rice were rinsed.

Oats: Oats are rich in soluble fiber, which has a cholesterol-lowering effect as well as the ability to help stabilize blood sugar levels.

Stone-ground whole wheat

Wheat berries: Wheat grains in their whole state

Whole grain

Whole wheat

Unlike the terms above, the following words on the ingredient list do not guarantee that whole grains are being used:

Multigrain: This means that the product contains a mixture of different types of grains but not necessarily whole grains. Consumers often confuse multigrain with whole grain.

Organic flour: This refers to the way the grain for the flour was grown and doesn't refer to whether the product is or isn't whole grain.

Semolina: Mostly used in pastas; may or may not be the whole grain

Wheat flour: May or may not be from the whole grain

Nutrition Facts Panel: Even if the product you are purchasing has a whole grain stamp, be sure to also look at the Nutrition Facts Panel for additional information. Pay close attention to the categories of **sugar, calories, fat, and fiber**.

It's worth noting that because whole grains include the germ, which is mostly fat, some wholegrain products (such as whole grain pasta) may be higher in fat than similar refined grain products, so don't be frightened away from a healthier whole-grain product if it contains a few grams of fat (you may see this reflected in the "calories from fat" section on your label). Remember that certain fats are healthy and important for you—check your label to be sure you're not getting saturated or trans fats accompanying your grains.

100% whole wheat: The word "wheat" alone is not enough to ensure that what you're buying is a nutritious food. This misleading term is found throughout your supermarket in the cereal, pasta, bread, and cookie (yes, cookie) aisles. You should be looking for "100% whole grain." "Whole wheat" could just mean that the wheat used is white; after all, white flour is wheat. The FDA has no set regulations for grain content. The FDA only has guidelines set for specific whole-grain flours and products such as breads and buns.

Wheat germ: Wheat germ is just that, the germ of the grain. Therefore, it is not a whole grain. Wheat germ does, however, have its health benefits. As mentioned earlier, the germ of a grain is rich in essential fatty acids as well as vitamins E and B.

Loopholes in Whole-Grain Labeling

- **"100% wheat."** This phrase means that the only grain contained in the product is wheat. The product could be processed and white flour, which you should avoid. The food may **not** actually contain *whole* wheat.
- **"Multigrain."** A word that means the product contains more than one type of grain. The food may **not** actually contain *whole* grains.
- **"Stone ground."** This term refers to grain that is coarsely ground and may contain the germ, but not the bran. Often refined flour is the first ingredient, **not** *whole* grain flour.
- **"Pumpernickel."** This is coarse, dark bread made with rye and wheat flours. It usually does **not** contain mostly *whole* grain flours.

Breakfast Foods

Consumer advocate groups often target ready-to-eat cereals, pointing to high sugar and sodium content and low fiber and healthy grain content. Although some types come close to candy in a box, lots of cereals have redeeming qualities, such as being fortified with vitamins and minerals, and they generally are paired up with a perfect partner, like a cup of skim or low-fat milk. Eating cereal, therefore, often means an intake rich in calcium and vitamin D (coming from milk) and, in some cases, fiber.

Grains make up the majority of foods eaten for breakfast. Breakfast is a vital part—often called the most important part—of your diet. Research studies have been conducted on the benefits of eating breakfast for children. Most studies show that breakfast helps children to increase their intake of calcium and vitamin D, as well as decrease their total caloric intake for the day. Those who skip breakfast are more likely to binge and snack on unhealthy food throughout the day to make up for the lack of calories in the morning. Although further research is needed, studies have indicated that eating breakfast in the morning may also help to improve cognitive function in children.

Cut Your Sugar Content in Half

Want to cut the sugar content of your cereal in half? If you (or your kids) can't resist some highly sugared cereals, try combining your sweet treat with a cereal that contains only 1 gram of sugar (check the sugar content on the label). Pour the contents of both boxes into a large bowl and mix them together. Then pour them back into their original boxes. Let's do the math: If one cereal has 1 gram of sugar and the other has 13, all we have to do is add them together and then divide by two. That'll bring your 13 grams-of-sugar bowl of cereal down to 7 grams.

If you really want to boost your breakfast choice, try adding a high-fiber cereal to the mix.

Fast Fact

Some types of cereal come close to candy in a box, but eating cereal can mean a higher intake of calcium and vitamin D (coming from milk) and in some cases, fiber. Kids in this country are in a calcium crisis, so the right cereal could provide profound benefits.

How to Shop for Cereal

The cereal aisle is one of the largest in the grocery store, and it seems like each brand of cereal has a claim on its label. Many cereals, even some that are good sources of whole grains and fiber, are also heavily processed and filled with sugar, fat, and additives, so choose wisely. If you take your kids shopping with you, try to teach them about not getting fooled by the cute characters on the colorful front of the box; it's what's inside that goes inside of them. If they're old enough to understand, the cereal aisle is a great place to compare Nutrition Facts Panels to pick healthier options.

Beware of health claims on packages promising to boost your immune system or unclog your arteries. Although there are many healthful ingredients in cereals, like soluble fibers, which can decrease the risk of heart disease, diabetes, and cancer, no one food is going to possess the cure for every ailments.

As an illustration, cereals that are low in saturated fat, cholesterol, and total fat and rich in soluble fiber (often cereals containing oat bran, rolled oats, whole oat flour) may link their product to decreased risk of heart disease. According to FDA regulations, in order to be able to make a statement linking heart disease to soluble fiber, the cereal must contain at least 0.6 gram of soluble fiber per serving. But remember—a bowl of cereal is just *one* component of a healthy diet, and 0.6 gram of fiber only makes a dent in the 30-plus grams you need each day.

According to the FDA, grain foods that are low in fat and are good sources of dietary fiber may legally contain a health claim related to a reduced risk of cancer. However, even these health claims must state that cancer is a "disease associated with many factors."

What to Look for on the Label

Carbohydrate: Whether hot or cold, whole-grain cereals contain more fiber, less sugar, and hunger-squashing complex carbohydrates. Be sure whole grains, including oats, barley, or brown rice, are mentioned first in the ingredient list. Be careful with granola-type cereals because although they may contain whole grains, they often also include lots of fat and added sugar.

Fat: You might not expect to see harmful fats lurking in cereal, and most manufacturers have eliminated partially hydrogenated oils (trans fats) from their ingredients, but check the ingredient list before buying cereal just to be sure.

Fiber: What does a high-fiber mean in terms of cereal? Try shooting for at least 5 grams or more per serving. Fiber is beneficial for proper bowel function and may aid in weight loss, cholesterol reduction, and blood glucose control.

Ingredient list: In general, the shorter the better. Whole grains should be at the top; sugars may appear as cane juice or molasses; and artery-clogging fats may be listed as partially hydrogenated fats.

Sugar: Cereals could contribute a significant source of sugar to your diet. Look for less than 5 grams of sugar per serving. Although you may not be scooping your spoon into the sugar bowl, remember that there is 1 teaspoon of added sugar per 4 grams of sugar. So a cereal with 16 grams of sugar per serving would contain about 4 teaspoons of sugar per serving.

If you are purchasing a cereal with fruit included (such as raisins) don't be turned off by a high sugar content. Fruits contain natural sugars, which increase the sugar content per serving of cereal (nutrition labels do not yet distinguish between natural and added sugars), but it's better to add your own fresh fruit instead of relying on sugary raisins for vitamins and minerals.

Fast Fact

The best cereals have whole grains listed as the first ingredient and at least 5 grams of fiber per serving. Sugar content should be 5 grams or less, and you should shoot for the shortest possible ingredient list.

Whole-Grain Cheat Sheet

- Look for products that list whole grain(s) as the first ingredient(s).
- Look for whole-grain products that contain at least 2 grams of fiber per serving, as wholegrain foods are rich in fiber.
- Look for products that display this health claim: "Diets rich in whole grain foods and other plant foods and low in total fat, saturated fat, and cholesterol may reduce the risk for heart disease and certain cancers." Such products must contain at least 51 percent whole grain by weight.
- Look for whole wheat pasta that lists whole wheat flour as the first ingredient. Most pasta is made from refined semolina or durum wheat flour.

Additive Alert: Be especially careful about these additives in grains

Acesulfame-K: This sweetener, sold under the brand names of Sunette or Sweet One, is often found in baked goods. Tests have shown that it may cause cancer in animals and therefore may increase cancer risk in humans.

Butylated hydroxyanisole (BHA): This chemical prevents oxidation and delays rancidity in foods that contain oil. Although it is potentially carcinogenic, it appears in hundreds of processed foods. Many breads, crackers, and snack foods contain BHA.

Olestra: Marketed under the brand name Olean, this synthetic fat is not absorbed by the body, and therefore can cause diarrhea, loose stools, abdominal cramps, and flatulence. Olestra also reduces the absorption of fat-soluble nutrients, including lycopene, lutein, and beta-carotene. Olestra is substituted for real fat in crackers and potato chips.

Partially hydrogenated and hydrogenated vegetable oils: These trans fats are linked with heart disease, breast and colon cancer, atherosclerosis, and elevated cholesterol levels. Look for them in processed foods like waffles and many baked goods as well as a variety of other products.

Potassium bromate: An additive used to strengthen bread dough and increase volume. It has been associated with causing cancer in laboratory animals.

Chapter 13

Just the Fats, Ma'am: Oils, Butter, Spreads, and Sprays

Fats

Finally, fats are getting a little respect.

For decades, Americans have fallen in and out of love with fats. Here's a news flash: We can't live without them. They are essential for our minds and bodies. The problem is we eat too much of them. Health professionals have been trying to get the word out that some fats should be avoided, while others should be an important part of our diets. For many consumers, it's hard to tell the difference.

The benefits and different types of fats are outlined in the first part of my book, but for a quick review:

- **Fats** are a great source of energy, providing 9 calories per gram.
- **Unsaturated (monounsaturated and polyunsaturated) fats** are beneficial for heart health.
- **Saturated fats** should probably be kept to a minimum although recent media buzz has these fats falling back in favor. Some say that they may not be as harmful as once believed, but that doesn't necessarily mean that they are good for us.
- **Trans fats** should be avoided altogether.
- **Essential fatty acids** are "essential" to the body because we cannot make them ourselves. Examples include omega-3 and omega-6 fatty acids.
- **Nonessential fatty acids** can be made in your body. An example is cholesterol; that's why even with a carefully cholesterol-controlled diet, some people have high cholesterol levels—they just manufacture a lot.
- **Conjugated linoleic acid (CLA)** are naturally found in dairy products and some meats. Researchers are finding potential links between CLA and decreased risk of certain cancers. Don't be surprised if you see this fat mentioned on more food labels in the near future.

Fast Fact

It would have served us better if "fats" were instead called "lipids." Although two-thirds of our population is overweight or obese, many of us fear the word "fat," assuming that if we eat any fat, we will get fat, thereby missing out on the benefits of healthy fats.

Let's look at some of the fats you'll see in the grocery store:

Butter, Spreads, and Margarine

Butter is made from cow's milk through the process of churning. Although many chefs could not live without its unsurpassed taste, butter has gotten a bad reputation because of its high saturated fat and cholesterol content. The food industry has taken advantage of this and thus created a variety of butter alternatives, including margarines and spreads.

The main advantage of **spreads** over butter is their vegetable oil origin. Vegetables oils have no cholesterol, and in fact, many of these spreads are now fortified with phytosterols (sterols and stanols), shown to help reduce the amount of LDL ("bad") cholesterol in your body. Phytosterols are naturally present in many plants, including vegetables, seeds, legumes, and vegetable oils. The FDA now allows health claims to appear on products containing plant stanols and sterols, which link these substances to the reduction of cholesterol and decreased risk of cardiovascular disease. According to the National Cholesterol Education Program's Adult Treatment Panel II, "Daily intakes of two to three grams per day of plant sterol/stanol esters will reduce LDL cholesterol by six to 15 percent." To achieve the needed 2 grams or more of plant stanols per day, in most cases, a serving size of 2 to 4 tablespoons per day is needed. These buttery spreads may contain any of the following types of vegetable oils: soybean, canola, sunflower, peanut, palm, corn, and olive oil. In addition, the spread will contain either water or milk.

You can expect to see plant sterols/stanols all over the store, appearing in salad dressings, bread and cereals, fruit juice, low-fat milk, and low-fat yogurt.

Margarine, on the other hand, may not contain cholesterol (because it is of vegetable rather than animal origin), but it undergoes a process called hydrogenation in order to turn it from a liquid to a solid state. This process creates trans-fatty acids, proven to be dangerous to your health. Margarine can also come without trans fats in the form of tub margarine. Margarine can contain the same amount of calories as butter, but you can also find reduced-calorie versions.

How to Shop for Butter, Spreads, and Margarine

There's a wide "spread" in how these products are displayed. Whether it's a tub, squeeze bottle, spray, or stick, it's important that you know what's inside the container. The bottom line is that if you're presently using trans-fat-laden shortening, and hard stick margarine. . . stop. If you need a spread for your toast, select one that is made with soft, non-hydrogenated vegetable oils, as listed below.

The USDA has set standards of identity for butter substitutes as follows:

Fat-free spreads: The fat content of this spread must be less than 0.5 gram per serving.

0 grams trans fats or trans fat free: This type of claim can be made if there is less than 0.5 gram of trans fats in your spread.

Margarine: Even if the label says 0 grams trans fat, don't put this product in your shopping cart before checking the ingredient list; if it contains partially hydrogenated fat, put it down and keep walking. You'll save both money and your heart.

Shortening: Usually in the form of vegetable shortening; this product is hydrogenated vegetable oil with a very extended shelf life as a result of the hydrogenation process. Shortening is technically a type of margarine; the difference is that shortening is 100 percent fat, while margarine also contains some protein and sometimes milk solids. I'd advise skipping this product, too.

Buttery spread: It must be made with liquid vegetable oils and contain 5 percent or less butter, with 5 grams or less saturated fat per tablespoon. In addition, buttery spreads may only have trace amounts of cholesterol.

Light buttery spread: A spread that contains no cholesterol, 0-2 grams of saturated fat, and is 50 percent lower in fat and calories than regular butter because it has less fat and more water.

Whipped butter: Whipped butter is whipped with air to make it light and fluffy and comes in tubs, making it an ideal table spread. Whipped butter has 30 percent fewer calories than solid butter and therefore less fat.

Salted butter: This butter contains almost one-half teaspoon of salt (or 1,000 mg of sodium) in a stick (8 tablespoons). If you're watching your sodium intake, you can use unsalted (sweet) butter instead. The shelf life of salted butter is longer than unsalted butter, though, as salt acts as a preservative. Salted butter can be stored for up to five months in the refrigerator and up to nine months in the freezer, whereas unsalted butter can be refrigerated for up to three months and frozen for up to five months.

European-style butter: Used throughout Europe, hence its name, and also known as raw cream butter, this product has 2 percent more milk fat than regular butter and is derived from fresh or cultured unpasteurized (raw) cream. Chefs often prefer this butter's richer taste and smoother texture when preparing baked goods and sauces.

Clarified butter: This type of butter has had most of its water and milk solids removed, which makes it a better fat to work with at high temperatures, as clarified butter has a higher smoke point than regular butter. Clarified butter (as well as ghee, which is heated longer than clarified butter to brown the milk solids and impart a nutty flavor) is almost 100 percent fat, thereby containing more fat and calories per teaspoon than butter, but may be better digested by those who are lactose intolerant because it contains almost no lactose.

What to Look for on the Label

Ingredients: Words you should steer clear of include **"hydrogenated"** and **"partially hydrogenated."** These words indicate the presence of harmful trans fats. You will see them in margarine and shortening packages. Research studies have continuously shown that trans fats increase the risk of coronary heart disease. Also pay attention to the type of vegetable oils used in margarines and spreads. Spreads can include any number of vegetable oils, one of them being peanut oil, so people with peanut allergies should pay particular attention.

Nutrition Facts Panel: This is where you can find out about the product's **trans fat**, **saturated fat**, and **cholesterol content**. As of 2006, all Nutrition Facts panels are required to list the amount of each of these fats. In addition to gram amounts, percent Daily Values are listed for saturated fats and cholesterol. There is currently no reference daily value for trans fats (but we know it should be zero); therefore, this percentage is not listed on food labels. Quick refresher course: 5 percent DV is low, so try to keep your saturated fat and cholesterol values at or below this number. A percent DV of 20 is high—don't go there in this category.

And also don't forget to **consider the calories**. These products are not calorie-free. As a matter of fact, some products provide the same calories as butter, so check the calories listed on the NFP to determine how much you can afford to use.

Fortification: Many butter substitutes are fortified with a variety of nutrients. Look for calcium and vitamin D fortification in buttery spreads. Fortification with plant stanols and sterols could help control cholesterol levels. Spreads may also be fortified with omega-3 and omega-6 fatty acids, but I recommend eating fish, ground flaxseeds, or walnuts instead of looking for your omegas here.

Trans fat claims: According to the FDA, a label can state "trans fat free" if there is 0.5 gram or less trans fats per serving size of the spread. Proceed with caution when it comes to portion sizes, as I've mentioned throughout the book. Free is not always free when it comes to this claim. Look at the ingredient label to see what type of oils are being used to replace trans fats. Palm oil (see below), a saturated fat, is a popular substitute.

Oils

How to Shop for Oils

Unsaturated fats: When choosing oils, your best options are unsaturated types, namely monounsaturated fats such as olive, peanut, and canola oils, and polyunsaturated fats such as vegetable oils like safflower, corn, soy, and cottonseed oils.) From a nutritional perspective, these are the "good" fats and, if used in place of other fats, can lower your risk of heart disease by reducing the total cholesterol and low-density lipoprotein (LDL) cholesterol levels in your blood. Like olive oil, canola oil has been connected with a decreased risk of coronary heart disease. The FDA has granted canola oil manufacturers the right to include a heart health claim on their labels:

Tropical oils: It seems we're coming full circle with tropical oils. I remember when manufacturers of cakes, pastries, and crackers were proud to write "no tropical oils" on the front of their labels when these saturated fats were found to be unhealthy. Trans fats in margarine and other processed foods replaced these fats, but in recent times, with trans fats being removed from foods, these tropical oils have shown their faces once again.

The major tropical oils are palm, palm kernel, and coconut oils. Although these oils are high in saturated fat, it is a different type than the saturated fat that's derived from animal products like meat, cheese, and butter. Some people believe that because they come from plants that their saturated fat content may not be as bad for health, and that tropical oils may benefit the immune system and actually improve cholesterol levels. If, for the most part, your diet is low in saturated fat and cholesterol (and contains no trans fats), tropical oils need not be totally avoided, as long as they aren't hydrogenated. However, even though palm, palm kernel, and coconut oils are vegetable sources, they are highly saturated fat and could increase LDL cholesterol, thereby increasing the risk for heart disease.

Perhaps the take-away message here is that tropical oils are a better choice than products that contain trans fats (hydrogenated fat), but it's still debated as to whether they should be put on your shopping list.

In general, oils are more prone to rancidity and spoilage than their solid counterparts. Fats high in saturated fat and trans fats increase a product's shelf life... but might shorten yours!

What to Look for on the Label

Although purchasing oil may seem simple, pay close attention to food labels when deciding what to purchase:

General Oils:

Unrefined oils: You will see "unrefined" on the label of many oils. This means that the oil has undergone a minimal amount of processing. This usually is the healthiest option. These oils generally are flavorful and rich in color (you will notice unrefined olive oils are greener or darker than their refined counterparts). These oils tend to be more prone to rancidity and spoilage.

Refined oils: These oils have undergone significant processing. They usually have a longer shelf life but tend to lose some nutritional value as well as flavor.

Olive Oils:

Extra virgin: Olive oils are differentiated by their acidity level. Extra virgin oils are derived from the first pressing of the olives and are lowest in acidity and richest in flavor and quality.

Virgin: This type of oil is one step down from extra virgin; it has undergone minimal processing and still has a number of nutrients that are present in the crude oil. For those who aren't used to the flavor of olive oil but still wish to take advantage of olive oil's nutritional benefits, this may be the best option.

Pure: Labels which state "pure olive oil" contain a mixture of refined and unrefined olive oil. They are usually lighter in color but more shelf stable than virgin and extra virgin oils. This may be a good oil to purchase for those who don't want the sharp flavor of olive oil or to use for cooking at higher temperatures.

Light: Contrary to popular belief, this label has nothing to do with calories or fat! Light simply refers to the color and aroma of the oil. Light olive oil is perfect when you don't want the flavor of the oil to be noticeable in a dish but you still want a healthier option than butter or other vegetable oils. Light equals lighter color and flavor, but not calories.

Cold pressed: Cold pressed means that the oil was not heated over a certain temperature (usually 80°F) during processing, thus retaining more nutrients and undergoing less degradation. Cold-pressing is a chemical-free process using only pressure, resulting in a higher quality of oil that is naturally lower in acidity.

First pressed: First cold pressed is of even higher quality than regular cold pressed, indicating that the oil was made with the first pressing of the olives.

Fat-Free Products

How to Shop for Fat-Free Products

For some people, the word "fat" on a box is synonymous with the words "do not enter." They'll take a pass on a food if it contains even the slightest amount of fat, even if the source of fat is healthy, such as canola or olive oil. But it's not just fat that can make you feel fat: If you eat more than you burn off of *any food*, you can gain weight, even if that food is bananas!

"Fat-free" on a label, however, certainly sells products, and for many consumers, this label justifies eating foods, like desserts, that people otherwise might have refrained from eating.

What to Look for on the Label

Calories: Fat-free is not calorie-free. Don't let labels fool you into thinking that a fat-free claim makes the product a calorie-free food.

Sugar: To compensate for a lack of taste once the fat is removed, manufacturers often add sugars. Although the fat grams may be listed as zero, don't walk out of the store without checking to see how many grams of sugar are in that product. Remember that 1 teaspoon of sugar contains 4 grams of sugar. Be aware that most carbohydrate-based foods, such as rice, pasta, fruits, and vegetables, are naturally free of fat.

Serving size: Labeling for fat-free foods is subject to the same FDA regulations as for trans fats. This means that something can be labeled "fat-free" if it has 0.5 gram or less fat per serving, and servings sure can add up!

Servings per container: If you chose to eat fat-free foods, eat them in moderation as you would any food, but don't think that the words "fat-free" guarantee weight loss.

Ingredient list: If it doesn't have fat . . . what does it have? If the product has a long list of ingredients, you may be better off with an item with more value and less additives (even if it contains a little fat).

Additive Alert: Be especially careful about these additives in fats

Brominated vegetable oil (BVO): This additive is used to stabilize the citrus oils so they don't separate out in the liquid. BVO has been linked to organ system damage, birth defects, and growth problems. Although it is considered unsafe by the FDA, it is still legal to use.

Butylated hydroxyanisole (BHA): This chemical prevents oxidation and delays rancidity in foods that contain oil. Although it is potentially carcinogenic, it appears in hundreds of processed foods. Butter and shortening may contain BHA.

Monosodium glutamate (MSG): For those who are sensitive, MSG can cause headaches, tightness in the chest, and a burning sensation in the forearms and the back of the neck, also known as "Chinese restaurant syndrome." If MSG is present, the food package must reflect it. Those who need to avoid MSG should avoid hydrolyzed vegetable protein (HVP), which may be listed on packages as "flavoring." MSG is commonly found in sauces and gravies.

Olestra: Marketed under the brand name Olean, this synthetic fat is not absorbed by the body and therefore can cause diarrhea, loose stools, abdominal cramps, and flatulence. Olestra also reduces the absorption of fat-soluble nutrients, including lycopene, lutein, and beta-carotene. Olestra is substituted for real fat in many products, such as crackers and potato chips.

Partially hydrogenated and hydrogenated vegetable oils: These trans fats are linked with heart disease, breast and colon cancer, atherosclerosis, and elevated cholesterol levels. The FDA banned partially hydrogenated oils in 2015 as they declared they are no longer generally recognized as safe. Still look for naturally-occurring hydrogenated oils in margarines, solid fats, and spreads as well as a wide variety of other products.

Propyl gallate: This preservative is used to prevent rancidity in fats and oils and has been linked to causing cancer. It appears in vegetable oil.

Chapter 14

Delightful or Destructive: Snacks and Desserts

I couldn't get through a day without snacks, and snacking should be an important part your day, too. You just need to know how to snack properly.

Snacks are the perfect speed bump to help stave off that ravenous need to devour your next meal. Snacks can keep your blood sugar levels and mood stable and help you stay alert and focused. The right snacks can even help you lose or maintain weight, but impulsively chosen snacks could pile on the pounds.

A recent report found that 90 percent of people snack, while only 75 percent eat breakfast and 88 percent eat lunch. Clearly, this is a popular subject.

If you think cookies, chips, ice cream, and candy when you're having a snack attack, think again. Those types of between-meal breaks will zap your energy instead of giving you a boost.

The key to smart snacking is to choose foods that add value and satiety to your diet. Your goal should be to pick snacks that are nutrient rich (high in vitamins, minerals, protein, whole grains, fiber, and healthy fats) and to limit those that are calorie-rich (high in calories, sugar, sodium, and fat—especially saturated and trans fats). A few tips regarding shopping for snacks:

Food group variety: Look for snacks that incorporate more than one food group, displaying a blend of protein, carbohydrate, and fat. Try to incorporate fruits and vegetables as much as possible; this will ensure the nutritional value and density of your snack.

Macronutrient (protein/carb/fat) variety: Snacks are meant to "hold you over" until your next meal. The best way to do this is to combine carbohydrates with protein. Carbohydrates should be high fiber whole grains as much as possible. The fiber that comes from the whole grains prevents you from feeling hungry quickly. Protein, as well as the good fats, increases your levels of satiety and helps you feel fuller longer.

Minimize the processing: Highly processed snacks are often filled with sodium, sugar, and calories. Not all processed foods are void of nutrients, but a more wholesome diet of less refined foods is preferable.

Watch portion sizes: If you're trying to watch your weight, snacks should consist of about 100 to 200 calories. For slim and physically active people, or for growing children, snacks may need to be higher in calories.

Fast Fact

The best snacks contain a combination of complex carbohydrates (whole-grain breads, crackers) and protein (low-fat cheese, nut butter) to help get you to the next meal while satisfying your body and your mind. Overeating snack foods will weigh you down rather than boost your mood and energy level.

Granola, Energy, and Meal Replacement Bars

How to Shop for Bars

Some stores dedicate a whole aisle to granola, energy, and meal replacement bars. Here's some labeling information that will help you decide which ones are best for you:

Granola bars have a health halo: people think that they're good for you, when many are not. Although whole grains, nuts, and protein may be added to the mix, you need to look more closely at other ingredients within. For some products, granola bar means candy bar.

Energy bars help get us through the day as we face our to-do lists that are longer than a toilet paper roll. Sometimes a "meal in a bar" is a convenient way to grab "something" instead of "nothing," but be sure the something is composed of the nutrients you'd otherwise be getting from a meal. Some energy bars have little nutritional value and wind up zapping energy instead of creating it, while others offer a solid combo of protein and fat (from nuts) and whole grain carbs (from oats, etc.) and some other carbs in the form of real fruit.

Meal replacement bars can provide a similar balance of nutrients as a meal, but the calories should be higher (250 to 350 per serving) than a snack bar, as should the nutrient content. Other foods, such as a glass of milk or a yogurt can be eaten along with the bar to boost nutrition. Don't make it a habit to replace meals—take the time to eat a meal, and in the meantime, take the time to read the label on your bar.

Beware of false claims and advertisements on any type of bar. These products were first promoted to athletes, promising power and endurance. I have seen bars with a label on the front that boasts "high protein," only to find a listing of just 1 gram of protein on the Nutrition Facts Panel on the back.

What to Look for on the Label

Added sugars: If you are buying a bar made with real fruit, the number of grams of sugar will be higher because of the natural sugars present in the fruit. Look for signs of *real* fruit, not artificially flavored hints of fruit. Glance farther down the label to the ingredient list to see if other types of sugar (such as cane juice), particularly found in bars filled with jellies or jams or coated with chocolate, are present.

Calories: Most granola and energy bars fall within the range of 100 to 200 calories per serving. Try to keep your calories in check, but don't forget to look at the rest of the label to be sure your body is getting value from the calories you're consuming.

Carbohydrates: A whole grain (like 100 percent whole wheat) should be one of the first items mentioned on the ingredient list. The presence of whole grains means that you're getting some fiber (try to get at least 2 to 5 grams of fiber per serving) to help keep you fuller longer and aid digestion.
You don't have to limit yourself to 2 grams—one of my favorite bars has 12 grams of fiber per serving.

Fat/saturated/trans fats: Look for 5 grams of fat or less per serving. Limit saturated to 1 gram or less per serving and avoid trans fats, listed as partially hydrogenated oils on the ingredient label.

Percent Daily Value: Many granola bars have added vitamins and minerals (such as calcium). Go for the most *valuable bars that are richest in important nutrients.*

Protein: Shoot for 4 (or more) grams of protein per serving. Protein will help sustain you longer by helping to squash hunger.

Sugar alcohols: Sometimes sugar alcohols (such as xylitol, maltitol, sorbitol, erythritol, and mannitol) are used instead of or in addition to sugar to keep the grams of sugar and calories lower. These products may raise blood sugar more slowly than real sugar, but they do contain calories and may cause a bloated feeling and other gastrointestinal issues.

Crackers

How to Shop for Crackers

There are so many types of crackers in the supermarket. Crackers can be a good source of whole grains, fiber, and trace minerals and vitamins, but they can also be a hidden source of sodium, fat, chemical additives, and empty calories. Some varieties have fillings (such as peanut butter or processed cheese) that add ingredients you're better off adding yourself, with a healthier, less processed version. Look for crackers that have short ingredient lists, with whole grains appearing first.

What to Look for on the Label

Carbohydrates: As with granola bars, read the label to see what's in your cracker. Eating crackers is a perfect way to up your intake of whole grains. Many brands use the whole grain stamp right on their packages, but don't stop at the stamp—check the other ingredients for added sugars.

Fat: Crackers can be a surprisingly high source of fat, and until recently, a significant contributor of harmful trans fats. Try to avoid those with saturated and trans fats, check the ingredient list to help you stay away from partially hydrogenated fats. Look for low-fat or fat-free options when possible, and try to walk past those with high-fat fillings.

Fiber: If you purchase whole-grain crackers, you'll notice the grams of fiber on the label may be higher than highly processed crackers made with white flour.

Serving size: See how many crackers are in one serving on the Nutrition Facts Panel. The serving size for some crackers is listed as 1 or 2, while others have servings of 23. Also, be sure to check how many servings are in the box and try to not eat out of the box to help you keep track of portion sizes and calories (especially while you're watching TV!).

Sodium: Crackers can be a major carrier of hidden sodium. And some—those topped with salt—are not so hidden. Look for the low-sodium or sodium-free options. Check the sodium content in terms of percent Daily Values on the Nutrition Facts Panel; try to keep this number below 5 percent. Crackers with cheese and peanut butter may be much higher in sodium and fat.

Cookies

How to Shop for Cookies

If only Cookie Monster had a sidekick called Veggie Monster. Would kids be asking for veggies as a snack after school instead of a plate of cookies? Well, perhaps that's asking too much, but if kids were greeted with a tray of cut-up fruit or vegetables and hummus or yogurt dip, I think they wouldn't mind replacing a cookie break with a break from cookies a little more often.

Cookies are a favorite snack for kids and adults alike. If accompanied by a tall glass of skim milk, the cookie side dish could make a delicious sometimes food. If cookies are your main-dish snack, then you're having dessert, not a healthy snack. They generally fall into the empty-calorie category, so read labels carefully to seek out the better ones.

The main ingredients in cookies are flour, fat, and sugar. It's the *types* and *amounts* of these ingredients that determine a cookie's nutritional value. Healthier varieties will include whole-grain flours (not just the white bleached kind), healthy fats (non-hydrogenated oils rather than butter or hydrogenated fats), and a limited amount of sugar (remember, 4 grams of sugar is equal to 1 teaspoon of sugar). These treats take up practically a full aisle in the supermarket, so save some time to compare package labels.

What to Look for on the Label

Added/refined sugars: Cookies are often made with refined or added sugars. You also may notice artificial sweeteners; manufacturers use them to lure you in with lower calorie and sugar scores. These products may be advertised as being "sugar-free" or "low-sugar" treats; remember, these terms do not necessarily mean low-calorie. Read the ingredient list to see what type of sweeteners you're getting. Artificial sweeteners and sugar substitutes still provide calories, and they're not safe for everyone.

Don't be fooled by ingredients like brown sugar, organic sugar, and raw sugar. These sweets are far from healthy, no matter how they are described.

Calories: Keep in mind, though, that purchasing whole-grain or oatmeal cookies doesn't mean you can eat an unlimited amount of them; sugar, fat, and calories should still be evaluated when making a decision about purchasing cookies.

Fats: When purchasing cookies, look on the ingredient label for healthier sources of fats, such as nuts instead of chocolate chips. Look on the Nutrition Facts Panel for the grams of fats and the breakdown of the types of fat (saturated and trans fat) you're getting. Try to pass up the cookies that contain partially hydrogenated fats (trans fats).

Grains: Although cookies are not really thought of as healthy foods, there are healthier options, such as those that are made from whole grains such as oats and whole wheat flour. Whole grains should be listed as one of the first, if not the first, ingredient on the ingredient list.

Serving size: There is no standard serving for cookies. I have seen some very deceptive labels down this aisle, with manufacturers listing a serving size as one cookie (when was the last time you ate just one?) to make all the numbers that follow down the label look good. With the new Nutrition Facts Panel coming to food packages soon, serving sizes should be more realistic. Until then, check the serving size before you start eating them out of the box.

Chips

How to Shop for Chips

Chips are extremely popular as a snack food, but not all chips are alike. If you read the food label to keep on top of the specific points mentioned below and if you're careful about what you dip your chip into (salsa rather than a fatty or salty dip), you might be able to actually find a healthy option. Baked chips are the best choice; low-fat chips come in second. Look for those made with nonhydrogenated oils (canola, soybean, sunflower, or olive oil) and those that provide whole grains, beans, seeds, and fiber. Whole-grain pretzels and popcorn are also good choices, but here, too, keep an eye on the sodium and fat contents.

What to Look for on the Label

Baked versus fried: Choose chips that are baked, not fried. Baked will most likely be lower in fat content, but that doesn't necessarily mean that they come with a health halo. As a matter of fact, I've seen some chips labeled "baked" and "all-natural" that have more sodium than fried chips.

Fiber: Check the fiber content on the label and try to choose products that are considered to be a "good source" of fiber, meaning that they provide at least 10 percent of the recommended daily value of fiber in one serving.

Ingredients: Choose chips made from whole grains, sweet potatoes, soy, beans, seeds, and other options that offer greater nutrient value than fried versions that are void of value. If the chips contain whole vegetables, you'll be assured of getting some fiber in your snack. Just be sure to read the label to see where on the ingredient list the vegetable is named: If it's mentioned at the end of a list of eight ingredients, don't count this snack as a serving of vegetables. Some veggie chips are not made from real vegetables but rather just a sprinkle of vegetable flour or powder.

Olestra: Olestra, also known as Olean, was the first noncaloric fat replacer, used in a host of favorite snack foods like chips, popcorn, crackers, and cheese puffs. It's basically made of table sugar and oil and is not digested or absorbed by the body. Although it is meant to give a rich taste and smooth texture to food without adding calories, it could add some unexpected gastrointestinal issues. In sensitive individuals, olestra-containing products can cause soft or loose stools and flatulence and other digestive issues (including one popularized in the media known as "anal leakage"), as well as prevent the absorption of essential fat-soluble vitamins. These unpleasant side effects may not occur if your portions are kept in check, but if you are able to watch your portion sizes, you're better off consuming a small amount of baked chips (*without* olestra) instead.

Serving size: "I'll bet you can't just eat one" was the tagline for a popular brand of chips when I was growing up. That's because chips are difficult to resist, making it hard to keep your hands out of the bag. When you're reading the calories on the NFP, don't forget to check the serving size. In some cases, unrealistic sizes like 8 to 10 chips can be listed as a serving, making the numbers that appear thereafter seem surprisingly low.

Sodium: If the sodium content looks low, check the serving size and servings per container. Remember to multiply each number on the NFP by the number of servings contained in the package. Shoot for less than 140 mg of sodium per serving size.

Healthy, Mood-Soothing, Perfect-Marriage, Snack-Attack Combos
Fresh vegetables dipped in hummus
Greek-style yogurt mixed with applesauce
High-fiber/low-sugar cereal with skim milk
Almond or peanut butter on whole-grain crackers
Part-skim cheese melted on whole-grain bread
Mixed unsalted nuts and dried fruit

Ice Cream and Frozen Yogurt

How to Shop for Ice Cream and Frozen Yogurt

There are so many delicious choices in the ice cream aisle. Ice cream is traditionally made with heavy cream, laden with saturated fat and cholesterol, and some premium types still contain as much fat per serving as a few pats of butter. But today there are many brands that are happy to let you know, via their labels, that they are "double churned," "slow churned," "light," and "fat and sugar free." They don't all taste the same, so you and your family will have to experiment (not a tough assignment) to see which one suits your needs and taste buds. Just don't forget that no matter which frosty treat you choose, your calories will climb if you add toppings like crumbled cookies, granola, or hot fudge.

Be sure to check labels of frozen desserts carefully, as the numbers listed on their packages could differ dramatically.

What to Look for on the Label

Added sugars: Although ice cream contains some natural sugar from the milk it's made with, check the ingredient list to see what other sugars are included, such as chocolate chips, candy, crunchy cookies, caramel, and sprinkles. A chocolate topping is usually high in fat and added sugar.

Artificial sweeteners: Frozen desserts that boast about not having as much sugar as their competitors have not come up with secret formulas to cut sugar without adding something else. Sugar substitutes like artificial sweeteners and sugar alcohols are added to keep calories down and keep table sugar at bay.

Calories: Choose a frozen dessert that has about 120 calories per serving.

Saturated fat/trans fat/cholesterol: Even if the brand you select has a red-heart endorsement from the American Heart Association, it doesn't necessarily mean that the product is in fact healthful. Check the label and steer clear of artery-clogging saturated fat and trans fat (partially hydrogenated fat). Zero grams of these fats would be best, but if your favorite brand has 1 to 2 grams of saturated fat, enjoy every smooth bite, but not every day. As with trans fats, zero is perfect.

Serving size: It's hard to resist this creamy treat once you've sunk your spoon into the cup, so pay attention to the amount that's listed as a serving size. Generally, one-half cup, which is not very big, is one serving.

Slow-churned/double-churned: These terms refer to a process called "low-temperature extrusion," which reduces the size of the fat globules and ice crystals in ice cream without compromising a creamy mouthfeel. This type of ice cream can be as low as half the calories of their full-fat frozen counterparts.

Here's the Scoop on Frozen Desserts

Ice cream: It must have at least 10 percent milk fat by volume; it may or may not contain eggs. **Frozen yogurt:** It doesn't taste like the yogurt that comes in the dairy section—it can be as sweet and creamy as ice cream and can be fat-free or low in fat. It contains dairy that has been cultured, and some even contain active (good) bacterial cultures, but check the label and don't assume it is low in calories.

Ice milk: It's like an ice cream but contains milk instead of cream. It's lighter and less creamy than ice cream and lower in fat content. It may or may not be high in sugar.

Nondairy dessert: Sorbet and ices contain little or no fat at all but may be loaded with sugar. Nondairy creamers used in some of these treats can be high in saturated and trans fats.

Sherbet: Similar to sorbet but also contains dairy (milk); it usually has a fruit component.

Additive Alert: Be especially careful about these additives in desserts

Acesulfame-K: Also known as Sunette or Sweet One, Acesulfame-K is often found in baked goods, chewing gum, and gelatin-type desserts. Tests have shown that this sweetener may cause cancer in animals and therefore may increase cancer risk in humans.

Artificial colors: Many foods are colored with combinations of synthetic dyes like Blue No. 2, Green No. 3, Red No. 40, and Yellow No. 5. Although the FDA banned Red No. 3 from many cosmetics and some foods because of its link to thyroid tumors in rats, it's still being used in maraschino cherries. The concern is that synthetic dyes cause cancer. Yellow No. 5 must be listed on ingredient labels to prevent allergic reactions, hives, a runny or stuffy nose, or breathing difficulties in people who are sensitive. Artificial colors have also been linked to hyperactivity in children. Such colors and dyes may be present in baked goods and candies.

Aspartame: Sold as NutraSweet or Equal, aspartame appears in diet (reduced-calorie) foods and may cause dizziness, headaches, epileptic-like seizures, and menstrual problems in those who are sensitive and has been shown to increase the incidence of brain tumors, lymphomas, and leukemia in rats. Individuals who have phenylketonuria (PKU) are unable to tolerate products containing this artificial sweetener. An accumulation of phenylalanine in the blood of a baby with PKU can result in mental retardation. All packaged foods that contain aspartame carry warnings.

Brominated vegetable oil (BVO): Brominated vegetable oil is found in gelatin desserts and some baked goods; it is used to stabilize the citrus oils so they don't separate out. BVO has been linked to organ system damage, birth defects, and growth problems. Although it is considered unsafe by the FDA, it is still legal to use.

Butylated hydroxyanisole (BHA): This chemical prevents oxidation and delays rancidity in foods that contain oil. Although it is potentially carcinogenic, it appears in hundreds of processed foods. Many pastries and snack foods (such as chewing gum and potato chips) contain BHA.

Olestra: Marketed under the brand name Olean, this synthetic fat is not absorbed by the body and can cause diarrhea, loose stools, abdominal cramps, and flatulence. Olestra also reduces the absorption of fat-soluble nutrients, including lycopene, lutein, and beta-carotene. Olestra is substituted for real fat in potato chips.

Partially hydrogenated and hydrogenated vegetable oils: These trans fats are linked with causing heart disease, breast and colon cancer, atherosclerosis, and elevated cholesterol levels. Look for them in cookies, cakes, pastries, and a wide variety of other food products.

Propyl gallate: This preservative is used to prevent rancidity in fats and oils and has been linked with causing cancer. It appears in vegetable oil, potato chips, and chewing gum.

Chapter 15

Drink to Your Health: Beverages

"Santé," "l'chayim," "salud"—no matter what language you speak, toasts are often blessings for good health. But when the beverage is the color blue and contains more sugar than a candy bar, that drink is nothing to cheer about. Most of us don't realize how important it is to drink properly. Although newsstand shelves are lined with magazines containing hundreds of food and diet stories, fluids rarely get the attention they deserve. Despite the knowledge that we need to consume more liquids, most Americans are not adequately hydrated.

Just think about your last physical exam: If you were lucky, your doctor asked you about your diet, and if you were tipping the scales, you may have been told to lose some weight. But when was the last time your health care provider asked you about how much fluid you were drinking?

Since water is the largest constituent of the human body, comprising about 60 percent of your body weight, it's time to lift your glass a little more often.

Juice

Although juice can be a significant source of sugar and calories, it is usually a healthier alternative to soda and other sweetened beverages. Some juices are linked with specific health benefits: Cranberry and blueberry juice may reduce the incidence of urinary tract infections; prune juice may relieve constipation; grape juice may reduce your risk of heart disease; and grapefruit and orange juice may reduce the severity of the common cold. Vegetable juice can help fill the gap in your diet for those veggies you just can't seem to fit into your busy day.

How to Shop for Juice

Through misleading labels and claims, some juice manufacturers make you feel like you couldn't live without them. These juices may be supplemented with extra vitamins and minerals, like vitamin D and calcium, as well as antioxidants, omega 3-fatty acids, fiber, herbs, and a host of other ingredients. Proceed with caution with these beverages, because you may get more calories and less benefit than you bargained for, and in some cases, you could be paying more money and taking more supplements than you actually need.

Numerous health claims on certain designer juices make it seem as if they'll provide you with superpowers. For instance, the seemingly magical juice made from the acai (pronounced ahsighEE) berry of the Amazon rain forest has been popping up in ads and stores all over the country. Consumers need to be warned about online companies and pyramid schemes related to selling these juices and other snake oil–like products. A great majority of these items contain misleading labels and are not government regulated.

Most of the buzz about these berry juices is based upon advertisements and testimonials and celebrity endorsements. If finding good health was as easy as finding a bottle of juice, the juice aisle in your supermarket would need traffic lights. Before you drink up, be sure to read the percent Daily Values of the food label carefully to be sure that you're getting the vitamins and minerals you're paying for.

What to Look for on the Label

Affiliation with health organizations: Some juices have statements on the back of their labels such as, "This product complies with the American Heart Association standards for low sodium." It's true that juice barely contains sodium, so that's not exactly a news flash. Choose fresh fruit instead of the juice and you'll get heart-healthy fiber, too. This type of claim is just a hook to get you to buy the product.

All-natural: Some beverages have this claim on the front of their labels. "All-natural" generally has the connotation that the food doesn't contain artificial ingredients and is minimally processed; however, this term is not regulated and carries more weight than it should.

Antioxidant claims: Many juices contain a health claim on the front of the bottle that represents a high antioxidant content. Antioxidants are substances or nutrients that protect cells against damage. Fruits and vegetables are naturally high in antioxidants, so don't be fooled—you would derive the same benefits plus more (fiber) by eating the whole fruit.

Contains/provides/good source of: These claims often appear on the front of juice bottles. According to the FDA, these claims can only be made if that ingredient is providing 10 to 19 percent of your Reference Daily Intake (RDI).

Fruit drink: This beverage is flavored water (no juice) with or without added nutrients or herbs.

Ingredients: Always look at the ingredients of the juice you are purchasing. Watch out for sources of added sugars, which are sugars that are supplied to a product during processing in addition to the natural sugar of the fruit itself. These sugars can appear as high-fructose corn syrup, dextrose, honey, sugar, corn syrup, corn sweetener, brown sugar, glucose, fruit juice concentrate, invert sugar, maltose, malt syrup, molasses, evaporated cane juice, raw sugar, sucrose, or syrup.

Juice: Anything labeled juice (such as apple juice or orange juice) has to be made from 100 percent fruit juice. If you are a purchasing a mixed blend drink, this, too, can be labeled 100 percent juice if each of the juices making up the drink is made from 100 percent juice. If you are going to purchase juice, the healthiest option in the juice aisle is 100 percent juice.

Juice cocktail, beverage, punch, or blend: These words on the product label indicate that the beverage you're purchasing has anywhere from 10 to 99 percent juice, but never 100 percent. The percentage of juice appears on the Nutrition Facts Panel on the product label. These beverages may contain some real fruit juice, sweeteners (such as sugar or high-fructose corn syrup), citric acid (to balance sweetness), and other ingredients (such as flavorings, color enhancers, and vitamins). They are not the best option and often provide more sugar than valuable nutrients. These products do, however, contain more nutrients than juice drinks.

Made from concentrate: All juices are required to say "made from concentrate" on the front label if their product contains any juice made in that fashion (most of the water content in the original juice has been removed, thereby making the juice more concentrated). Once the juice is concentrated, it is transported to its manufacturing location, where water is added, and as long as there is no change in the juice (aside from water being removed and replaced), the label can state that the juice is 100 percent juice from concentrate.

Made with artificial flavors: According to the FDA, food labels must contain this statement if they use substances that do not come from an animal or a plant in order to impart flavor. Usually fruit juices do not boast about his claim, as health-conscious consumers are looking for pure and natural ingredients. Check the ingredient list to be sure you know which flavors are being added.

Made with natural flavors: According to FDA regulations, food labels can have the phrase "made with natural flavors" if the flavors have been produced from a plant or an animal source directly. This includes spices, fruits, vegetables, yeast, herbs, bark, buds, roots, leaves, and so on. The term "natural" is still confusing and sometimes misleading when it comes to flavorings.
Artificial ingredients *must* be labeled as such, to help you determine whether the food is only made with natural flavorings or made with natural *and* artificial flavorings (in which case it must be indicated). And keep in mind that the term 'organic' is not synonymous with 'natural,' but organic foods can have natural flavorings (nonorganic) as long as the products are 95 percent or less organic. This means that flavorings can be present in up to 5 percent of the food's ingredients to be in compliance with the National Organic Program.

The USDA's Food Safety and Inspection Service defines "natural" as "a product containing no artificial ingredient or added color and is only minimally processed (a process which does not fundamentally alter the raw product) may be labeled natural." Most foods labeled natural, including their flavorings, are not subject to government controls beyond the regulations and heath codes.

Made with real juice: This type of claim is particularly enticing to today's organic-minded, health-conscious shoppers, and is often used to lure them in to buy their products. Sadly, many beverages that carry this claim may contain as little as 3 percent fruit juice. Always turn the bottle around and look at the Nutrition Facts Panel. Above the serving size, at the very top of the label should be the percentage of real fruit juice contained within. Oftentimes this is written in very small print, and because it isn't technically part of the NFP (not included in the box), many consumers miss this crucial information.

Organic: Many juices wear "organic" labels on the front of their bottles, but even if a juice is organic, it doesn't necessarily mean that the juice is low in calories or sugar. In fact, even if a juice is organic it doesn't necessarily mean that it's 100 percent juice! "Organic" describes the way in which a food is grown; it does not reflect its nutritional value. Organic produce is grown without synthetically compounded fertilizers, pesticides, herbicides, hormones, medicated feed, or antibiotics or chemicals used in food processing. It's the production, not necessarily the product, that's different.

Not from concentrate: This juice is sold ready-to-drink and is the closest to fresh juice. Juice that isn't made from concentrate is often described as "fresh squeezed" and will have a shorter shelf life than juice made from concentrate. It will state "not from concentrate" on its label.

Reconstituted juice: Oftentimes when you look at the ingredients label of juice, the first ingredient is "reconstituted _____ juice." This simply means that the juice was first concentrated (water removed) and then the water was put back into the juice.

Tea

Tea is becoming an incredibly popular beverage in the American diet, appearing in colorful boxes and carrying enticing labels. You'll find teas that profess to calm your mood, ease constipation, help you feel more awake, soothe you to sleep, boost your immune system, and help you speak with an English accent (just kidding about that last one). These claims are not always clearly written on the box but instead are reflected in the tea's name (such as Tummy Tamer, Smooth Move, Get Regular, Sleepytime, Throat Coat, and so on).

How to Shop for Tea

Tea producers have taken advantage of the inherent benefits of antioxidants and have done a great job of packaging and promoting their products, especially when it comes to the sale of iced teas. Although drinking tea has many benefits, including promoting bone health, protecting the immune system, aiding digestion, and keeping us hydrated, not all teas are harmless. Proceed with caution with teas that add supplements (vitamins and minerals) and herbs that could interfere with other medications or supplements you may be taking. Some teas have added ingredients that provide no greater benefit than just drinking water. You might need to drink a case of tea made with St. John's wort, an herb used to ease depression, to be equivalent to 1 pill containing the same herb. But since the amount of the herb added is not standardized or identified specifically, you'd never be able to figure that out.

Most herbal teas include the type of leaves used on the ingredient list. The great majority of these beverages are caffeine-free, but be sure to check the label because some do contain caffeine.

Types of Tea

Although the tea aisle is expanding by leaps and bounds, all teas come from the same plant *(Camellia sinensis).* Here is a description of the varieties:

Black: Black tea is what we commonly think of when we refer to tea. Black tea leaves oxidize as they are being exposed to warm, dry air, causing the leaves to darken, and are then fired, bringing out their full-bodied flavor.

Oolong: These leaves are only partially oxidized (as opposed to fully oxidized for black tea) before they are fired.

Green: The leaves used for green tea are the same as those that make black and oolong teas, but they are either steamed or pan-fired right after being picked rather than being oxidized. Green tea contains powerful antioxidants called polyphenols, which protect the cells in your body.

White: These tea leaves are picked from buds that are newer than those used for green tea. The leaves are air-dried, which allows them to retain their delicate flavor as well as potent antioxidants.

Red tea: This tea is made from the needle-like leaves of the rooibos plant. It is caffeine-free and contains antioxidants as well as traces of other nutrients (such as calcium and zinc).

Herbal tea: Herbal teas come in a wide variety of types and are often made not just from the leaves, but also the flowers, roots, bark, and seeds of one or more plant. Though nearly all types of herbal tea are naturally caffeine free, there are a couple of exceptions; certain green teas contain caffeine, and Guarana and Yerba mate' teas contain guaranine and mateine, respectively, that are similar in chemical makeup to caffeine. People who are sensitive to caffeine may need to avoid these products. Check the label for the word "decaffeinated" if you want to avoid caffeine. The great majority, however, are caffeine-free.

Chai: This beverage is made from black tea with a blend of several spices, generally served with milk and a sweetener such as honey or sugar.

> **Fast Fact**
>
> Don't assume that your herbal tea doesn't contain caffeine. If you need to restrict caffeine, it should say "caffeine-free" or "decaffeinated" on its label.

What to Look for on the Label

Antioxidants: Antioxidants provide protection to our cells by delaying or preventing damage caused by free radicals. They are believed to reduce risk of cancer and heart disease, slow down the aging process, and improve overall health. According to the FDA, to claim that a product is "high in antioxidants" on the label, the product must contain 20 percent or more of the Daily Reference Value (DRV) or Reference Daily Intake (RDI) of the specific antioxidant per serving. One little glitch is that not all antioxidants have DRVs or RDIs; daily levels have been established for some antioxidants, such as vitamins C and E, but not all. The FDA also has set a special rule for antioxidants such as beta-carotene, which the body converts to vitamin A: Products high in betacarotene can base claims on the DRV/RDI for vitamin A. Products that don't meet the 20 percent threshold but do provide at least 10 percent of the DRV/RDI per serving can claim to be a "good source" of an antioxidant.

Enhanced: Look at the ingredient label carefully and choose teas that contain the fewest amount of ingredients; herbal supplements, vitamins, and minerals, which some teas are fortified with, may be overstepping your needs.

Flavonoids: Flavonoids are a group of compounds found in plants and plant-based foods that that bolster the antioxidant defenses in cells and may lower the risk of certain diseases like cancer and heart disease. These compounds are often listed right on the package and/or on the individual packet of tea. Many consumers don't even know what antioxidants or flavonoids are, yet they feel comfort in seeing these words listed on their labels because of the perceived health benefits. In addition to tea, flavonoids are also found in apples, chocolate, grapes, and wine.

Good source of antioxidants: Must contain 10 to 19 percent of DRV or RDI per serving.

High in antioxidants: Must have 20 percent or more of the Daily Reference Values or RDI per serving.

Nutrition Facts Panel: Always look at the sugar content on the NFP as well as serving size and serving per container. Iced teas can be loaded with sugar and calories. Opt to choose the tea with the least amount of sugar, keeping in mind that every 4 grams of sugar is equal to one teaspoon of sugar. Artificially sweetened teas may represent a better option for people trying to control their weight or sugar intake, as for those individuals that have diabetes. Overall, try to choose a tea that's made of. . . tea, period.

Coffee

Coffee is something that seems to appear on both "good" *and* "bad" lists. Studies have shown that coffee can decrease your risk of developing diabetes, Parkinson's disease, asthma, and headaches as well as enhance athletic endurance. Coffee beans are rich in health-supporting antioxidants. For some, caffeine increases alertness and aids in concentration, whereas for others, the opposite is true, causing a jittery, nervous, uncomfortable feeling and gastrointestinal distress. Caffeine should be used with caution when it comes to selecting sources of hydration, as it has a dehydrating effect.

How to Shop for Coffee

Whether you buy your coffee in a giant superstore or a tiny specialty store, you'll find a variety of brands, flavors, types, and grinds. You will also notice certification labels on coffee that tell you where your beans came from as well as information about the coffee growers.

What to Look for on the Label

Bird-friendly/shade grown: Other labels you may find on your bag of coffee include the birdfriendly label, which meets all the standards set by the Smithsonian Migratory Bird Center, a label specifically stating that the coffee is shade grown (minimum 40 percent shade), organic (must be USDA certified organic), and grown without synthetic chemicals. Shade-grown coffee, in contrast to coffee produced by conventional sun-grown methods, provides food and shelter for songbirds as well as other animals and plants. Trees help maintain soil quality, and they also yield natural mulch, thereby diminishing the need for chemical fertilizers.

Decaffeinated: Although you may see the word "decaffeinated" on the label, decaffeinated coffee does contain a small amount of caffeine (6 mg caffeine per 10-ounce cup as opposed to 260 mg for caffeinated coffee).

Fair trade: This phrase, often seen on coffee labels these days, means that the coffee was purchased for a fair price directly from the coffee grower.

Organic: Organic refers to the way a product is grown and processed. When purchasing organic coffee, look for the USDA Organic seal, which will appear on coffees that are at least 95 percent organic. "certified organic" means the item was grown according to strict standards. Certification includes inspections of farm fields and processing facilities, detailed record keeping, and periodic testing of soil and water to ensure that growers and handlers are meeting the standards that have been set. Keep in mind, however, that buying organic coffee does *not* mean it is locally grown.

The Rainforest Alliance: The Rainforest Alliance label assures consumers that the coffee they're purchasing came to their home via practices carried out according to a specific set of criteria balancing "ecological, economic and social considerations." The Rainforest Alliance label also ensures that coffee farmers are paid at fair wages.

Fast Fact

For every cup of coffee you have, you should drink a cup of water. Caffeine should be used with caution when it comes to selecting sources of hydration, as it could have a dehydrating effect.

Soda

Sodas and other sweetened carbonated beverages are staples in the American diet, displacing other, healthier, beverages. The average can of soda can is equal to one can of water with ten packets of sugar in it.

How to Shop for Soda

What I'd really like to say is that when it comes to shopping for soda . . . don't. But since I know that millions of people all over the globe are buying this sweet stuff, we need to address the issues. If you drink soda, do so in moderation, whether it is made with sugar or artificial sweeteners. Soda has no nutritional value and it often replaces more nutritious beverages; it should be looked upon as a "sometimes" food rather than a staple. Check your food labels carefully and compare products, paying attention to grams of sugar and the percent Daily Value of nutrients within a soda. (Let me save you some time . . . there's no value.)

Fast Fact

How much soda should you shop for each day? None. Each 12-ounce can of soda is equivalent to a can of water with ten packets of sugar mixed in it.

If soda is your favorite treat, save it for restaurants and special occasions.

What to Look for on the Label

Caffeine: Many sodas, particularly colas, contain caffeine. Sodas have less caffeine per serving than coffee (45 mg per 12-ounce can as opposed to 260 mg per 10-ounce cup of coffee), but drinking a few cans a day can negatively affect your health. There are many decaffeinated sodas these days, so check the front of the label.

High-fructose corn syrup (HFCS): HFCS is a sweetener derived from corn and is used in soft drinks (and a vast array of processed foods) across the globe. It provides the same calories as sugar and acts in the same way, providing empty calories of no value. Although this product is often bashed by the media, basically, it's no better or worse than plain old added sugar. Both should be avoided when possible, especially when they are in the form of a calorie-loaded liquid.

Very low sodium: Sodas now can have a "very low sodium" claim on the Nutrition Facts Panel. Although legally the sodium content of most sodas is low enough to fall into this health claim category, that doesn't make soda a health food.

Water

Water is essential for every human being. It contains no calories, no sugar, no sodium, and no artificial sweeteners, and there's no reason to not drink it. Specific populations, in particular the elderly, have increased needs for water due to a decreased ability to detect thirst with age. Although you can get water free of charge from your tap, many brands of bottled water claim they are healthier, cleaner, and better than tap water, and many are also enhanced with vitamins and minerals. There is some controversy as to whether bottled water is preferable to tap water; in some locations, tap water has an unacceptable taste. In New York City, where I come from, tap water couldn't be better! Although tap water has its share of problems, like the potential for contamination and food-borne illness, these problems are fairly rare. A home filtration system will take care of the majority of any issues.

Bottled water is regulated by the Food and Drug Administration (FDA) as a packaged food product, and it must adhere to the FDA's extensive food safety, labeling, and inspection requirements. Bottled water is also subject to state regulations. By law, FDA standards for bottled water must be at least as stringent and protective of public health as standards set by the U.S. Environmental Protection Agency (EPA) for public water systems. There are many varieties of flavored and enhanced waters being sold in supermarkets and grocery stores; they are often a source of unnecessary calories and sugar and may contain other ingredients, such as caffeine. Soda water, seltzer water, and tonic water are regulated differently; they are classified as soft drinks. Be sure to check the label on any water you purchase because you may be surprised to find sugar, sodium, or caffeine added.

How to Shop for Water

Some brands state the source of bottled water on their label, mentioning whether the water is derived from public or private water sources, while others list this information on their Web sites rather than on the bottle.

What to Look for on the Label

Artesian water/artesian well water: This is bottled water from a well that taps a waterbearing underground layer of rock or sand in which the water level stands at some height above the top of the aquifer.

Enhanced/flavored waters: If you are buying flavored or enhanced water, it's important to check the Nutrition Facts Panel and the ingredient list to pay attention to what might be added to your beverage. There are flavored waters that have subtle flavorings added to include an essence of flavor without any additional calories or artificial ingredients. Carefully check your labels, though, for calories, added sugars, artificial sweeteners, and even caffeine. You should also examine the vitamin and mineral content carefully. Waters enhanced with vitamins may provide more than 100 percent of your DRIs for specific vitamins, depending on the serving size. Receiving more than the necessary amount of vitamins and minerals can be harmful for people suffering from some conditions.

Mineral water: Mineral water, by definition, contains more than 250 parts per million (ppm) of a mineral substance. It has the same proportion of minerals and trace elements as the original underground source of the water; no other minerals can be added. Mineral water generally has no calories.

Purified water: Water produced by distillation, deionization, or reverse osmosis may be labeled as purified bottled water. Other names for purified type of water may include "distilled water," "deionized water," and "reverse osmosis water."

Sparkling water: Sparkling water contains carbonation resulting from the introduction of carbon dioxide. Bottled sparkling water may be labeled as "sparkling drinking water," "sparkling mineral water," and "sparkling spring water." Sparkling water can be plain (seltzer), flavored, or enhanced with nutrients. Generally speaking, sparkling water is free of calories, but you can never be too sure: Check the calories and sugar on the NFP to see if any sugar has been added.

Spring water: Spring water comes from an underground formation from which water flows naturally to the surface of the earth. Spring water must be collected only at the spring or through a hole tapping the underground formation feeding the spring.

Well water: Bottled water from a hole that is bored, drilled, or otherwise constructed in the ground that taps the water aquifer.

Sports Drinks

When my boys played Little League, there were oceans of colorful bottled sports drinks sitting next to each child on the bench, even though these kids barely got any exercise.

Whether you actually need sports drinks depends on the length of your workout, the type of exercise you're doing, and how hard you're working. The benefits of these drinks, aside from replacing lost body fluids (hydration), are that they contain electrolytes (important minerals that regulate fluid balance and transmit nerve or electrical impulses), like sodium and potassium, both of which should be mentioned on the label. These fluids are also a source of carbohydrates and fuel for your brain and muscles. Research has shown that that for exercise lasting anywhere from sixty minutes to several hours, drinking sports beverages could boost endurance and performance.

How to Shop for Sports Drinks

There are a few factors to consider when looking at sport drinks, including the type of carbohydrates in the product and the concentration of carbohydrates and electrolytes. A beverage with a 6 percent carbohydrate solution (about 14 grams of sugar per 8 fluid ounces) optimizes sweetness, stomach emptying, rapid fluid absorption, and energy delivery to the exercising muscles. Most credible sports drinks are formulated to meet this recommendation. Beverages containing more than 8 percent carbohydrate tend to be too sweet, increase the likelihood of an upset stomach, and cause a slower absorption of fluid.

The take-home message is that, except for fructose, the kind of carb doesn't matter as much as the carbohydrate concentration; therefore, the more sugar, the more slowly it will be absorbed.

It's also important to pay attention to the size of the bottle, and remember that the numbers on the label represent the serving listed, not the entire contents. As far as how much of a sports drink to guzzle, the American College of Sports Medicine suggests, "1 ½ to 4 cups per hour (more if you have heavy sweat losses) will provide you with both the fluid and carbs you need for endurance." This suggestion could vary greatly, however, depending upon the athlete's personal genetics and the weather conditions. In any event, it's also important to remember to drink prior to and during exercise to keep your body properly hydrated.

Not everyone needs sports drinks: A cup of skim milk provides 12 grams of sugar, 127 mg of sodium, 407 mg of potassium, plus other valuable nutrients. For the average person doing moderate exercise, this may be a better drink of choice. Don't let a picture of someone climbing up Mt. Everest convince you to buy a beverage—turn the bottle over to get the facts.

What to Look for on the Label

Caffeine: Caffeine in sports drinks can boost performance and endurance for some people but cause the jitters and stomach upset for others.

"Energy": Everyone longs for endless energy, and manufacturers want you to believe you can get it in a sports drink. Marketing hype is often offered in the form of caffeine and sugar, both of which may provide you with quick but not lasting energy. The best way to get energy is to get enough sleep and eat the right foods, and you won't find this in a bottle in the supermarket.

Potassium: During two to three hours of hard exercise, you could lose 300 to 800 mg of potassium at about 80 to 100 mg potassium per pound of sweat. One cup (8 ounces) of a typical sports drink provides 32 mg of potassium. As a frame of reference, one cup of skim milk has 400 mg and one banana provides 500 mg of this important mineral.

Sodium: Sodium is an electrolyte lost in sweat. The sodium in sports drinks helps fluids get absorbed in your intestines, and its positive effect on flavor promotes proper hydration during and after exercise. Usually you'll find about 100 mg of sodium per 8 ounces.

Sugars: Sources of carbohydrate typically include sucrose (from beet or cane), glucose, fructose, corn syrup solids, high fructose corn syrup, maltose, and maltodextrins (sometimes called glucose polymers). Drinks containing mostly or only fructose are not recommended because fructose is absorbed more slowly than other sugars, resulting in a slower absorption of water and potentially leading to gastrointestinal distress.

Milks

Although some would say that beverages made from plants are not technically 'milks, 'these beverages are here to stay. Some provide valuable nutrients and they play an important role in the diet for those with lactose intolerance and for those who just don't do dairy.

In general, if you're looking to boost bone-building, it's best to choose a plant milk that's fortified with calcium and vitamin D and be sure to shake it well before drinking since these nutrients can settle to the bottom of the container. Unlike dairy milk, almond and soy milks both provide fiber, a nutrient important for gut health and for providing a moving experience.

Almond milk is naturally free of cholesterol, saturated fat, and lactose. Many brands of almond milk are fortified with calcium and vitamin D. Since almonds are high in protein, it might surprise you that almond milk has 1 gram of protein. Most of us get plenty of protein in our daily diets, so if you enjoy almond milk's tasty, nutty and satisfying flavor, you can pair it with other protein-rich foods and take advantage its versatility as an ingredient in recipes such as soups, smoothies and sauces.

Soy milk comes in many different versions including low fat, full fat, calcium-fortified, and flavored, just to name a few. If you're looking to boost bone-building, it's best to choose a soy milk that's fortified with calcium and vitamin D, and be sure to shake it well before drinking since these nutrients can settle to the bottom of the container.

Soy milk is a good alternative for those who have dairy allergies. Although soy milk is also rich in protein, flavored types tend to contain less than those that are unflavored.

Rice milk is made from a combo of partially milled rice and water. Although it has a sweetness and comes in a variety of flavors, it barely contains any protein. It is, however, the least likely of any milk to trigger an allergic reaction.

Hemp milk has a flavor similar to almond milk with a nutty, creamy finish. It is derived from hemp seeds that are rich in the plant-based omega-3 fatty acid, alpha-linolenic acid (ALA).

Although it's not as easy for the body to derive benefits from plant sources of omega-3s as it is from other sources like fish, ALA is beneficial in reducing risks of heart disease and inflammation. Since hemp milk is higher in fat content than other milk alternatives, you may need to keep portions in check.

Coconut milk is more like cream than milk and often gets confused with its lower-calorie relative, coconut water. Sweetened versions can pack almost 450 calories per cup of which 380 calories is saturated fat. Lighter versions are available, providing 60 percent less calories and fat that the original version.

Additive Alert: Be especially about these additives in beverages

Acesulfame-K: Acesulfame-K (also known as Sunette or Sweet One), is often found in soft drinks. Tests have shown that this sweetener may cause cancer in animals and therefore may increase cancer risk in humans.

Artificial colors: Many foods are colored with combinations of synthetic dyes like Blue No. 2, Green No. 3, Red No. 40, and Yellow No. 5. Although the FDA banned Red No. 3 from many cosmetics and some foods because of its link to thyroid tumors in rats, it's still being used in maraschino cherries. The concern is that synthetic dyes cause cancer. Yellow No. 5 must be listed on ingredient labels to prevent allergic reactions, hives, a runny or stuffy nose, or breathing difficulties, in people who are sensitive. Artificial colors, which are found in some soft drinks and fruit drinks, have also been linked to hyperactivity in children.

Aspartame: Sold as NutraSweet or Equal, aspartame appears in diet soft drinks and may cause dizziness, headaches, epileptic-like seizures, and menstrual problems in those who are sensitive and has been shown to increase the incidence of brain tumors, lymphomas, and leukemia in rats. Individuals who have phenylketonuria (PKU) are unable to tolerate products containing this artificial sweetener. An accumulation of phenylalanine in the blood of a baby with PKU can result in mental retardation. All packaged foods that contain aspartame must carry a warning.

Caffeine: This stimulant can cause nervousness, irritability, nausea, gastrointestinal upset, and insomnia, and it may worsen fibrocystic breast disease in some women. Since caffeine may also interfere with reproductive health and potentially affect a growing fetus (low birth weight), the FDA issued the following warning: "Pregnant women should avoid caffeine-containing foods and drugs, if possible, or consume them only sparingly." Caffeine has also been associated with hyperactivity in children. Caffeine is considered to be a drug and may be addictive, yet it is added to many foods, including soda and enhanced waters. Coffee, tea, and chocolate naturally contain caffeine.

Monosodium glutamate (MSG): For those who are sensitive, MSG can cause headaches, tightness in the chest, and a burning sensation in the forearms and the back of the neck, also known as "Chinese restaurant syndrome." If MSG is present, the food package must reflect it. Those who need to avoid MSG should avoid hydrolyzed vegetable protein (HVP), which may be listed on packages as "flavoring." MSG is may be hidden in certain iced tea mixes, sports drinks, soft drinks, and drinks made with protein powders.

Saccharin: Packaged as Sweet'N Low or SugarTwin, this artificial sweetener has been linked to cancer in laboratory animals. It was banned by the FDA in 1977; however, due to popular demand, Congress overrode the FDA's decision and exempt saccharin from regular food-safety laws. Saccharin is found in some diet beverages.

Chapter 16

Super Shopping Lists

Very early on in this book, I confessed that I love going food shopping. And now that I've shown you how to read (and not be fooled by) a food label, it's time for you to go shopping. You don't have to memorize any facts and figures—just take this book along with you into any supermarket (because the tips within these pages are not linked to any particular store or product) and fill your cart with delicious, healthy choices for you and your family.

But before you step out the door...remember to bring a shopping list. Whether you have a list or not can affect your entire shopping experience. Countless studies have shown that making a list ahead of time is the best way to avoid over-shopping, overspending, and, ultimately, overeating.

In many cities, with the use of computerized home shopping, you can stock your cabinets without ever leaving the comfort of your home. These services provide online shopping lists that include prepared meals as well as make-your-own shopping lists that you can save on their site for quick reference and future use. If online shopping is not your thing, but you can't get to the store to pick out your own groceries, some stores allow you to fax in your order and for a nominal fee have your groceries delivered to your door.

Fast Fact

Bringing a shopping list with you to the store can save you time as well as countless dollars and calories a year.

I have attached my **Ultimate Shopping List** to the end of this chapter so you can navigate the aisles of the supermarket and stock your pantry, fridge and freezer with healthful foods. There are many online shopping lists available as well, but just a word of caution—these lists may contain some unhealthy foods as well. My hope is that by reading my book you can sift through these lists and choose the healthiest options, thus make your shopping experience easier. And note that several of these sites may display advertisements from companies selling their products: Just ignore the flashes and go right to the shopping list. Save your purchases for the supermarket.

Here are some general guidelines before you go food surfing:
- Think about the foods your family likes to eat and compare your preferences to my Ultimate Grocery Shopping List to figure out how to adapt it to your particular needs.
- Print out my Ultimate Grocery Shopping List and highlight the items on the list to compile your own "master list." You can even copy this list, store it in your computer and keep it on the countertop or under a magnet on the fridge for every food shopping trip. Having your list accessible will enable you to circle items as needed or as you remember them. This will prevent you from not having enough of some items and from duplicating the ones you already have. Arrange this list according to the layout of the store you shop in most frequently to avoid needing to backtrack.

- Check with the registered dietitian nutritionist or manager at your supermarket to see if the store has a website that displays their own shopping list. Many big chains have helpful guides available as well.
- Plan ahead and shop for a few meals at a time so you don't have to go to the store too often.
- Although you've probably heard this a million times...*don't go shopping when you're hungry!* You'll ending up buying much more than you need.
- Try to stick to the list. I know this is easier said than done, but your wallet will thank you for it.

Shopping Lists and Where to Find Them

BetterThanDieting.com

When you sign up for my free Better Than Dieting weekly news digest, you'll get my super supermarket shopping guide to help you fill your fridge and pantry with staples you can rely on. I'll walk you down the aisle so that you can feel confident (instead of confusion) when you walk into any food store, any where. And let's connect on social media for ultimate tips on how to find the healthiest food for you and your family. I'd love to hear from you on Instagram (@bonnietaubdix), Twitter (@eatsmartbd), Facebook (Bonnietaubdix.RDN) and Pinterest (@bonnietaubdix).

Supermarket Savvy

www.supermarketsavvy.com or
www.supermarketsavvy.com/catalog_educator/product_detail.asp?product=8

Supermarket Savvy's Brand-Name Shopping List is a wonderful resource for consumers. It provides you with information about almost every food item you'll find in the store; a check mark signifies low sodium, and an X signifies high fiber. The Web site divides your foods into the aisles you'd commonly find in a regular supermarket: bread, meats and seafood, seasonings, fats and oils, beverages, snacks, and so on. It also gives you a portion size for specific foods, as well as fat content. Supermarket Savvy allows you to create your own shopping list by checking off options from different aisles and placing them in your virtual shopping cart. This is a comprehensive, credible resource.

RD411

www.RD411.com

This site is unique in that it provides a wealth of information written by registered dietitians, the nutrition experts. The patient education section has more than four hundred handouts on almost every nutrition topic, including shopping lists to guide you through the supermarket aisles via brand comparisons as well as general strategies. One of this site's philosophies is that one of the first steps to eating healthy is to fill your home with nutritious foods so you don't reach for empty calories. Other articles available discuss caffeinated beverages, reading food labels, shopping on a budget, snack ideas, controlling calories, and much more.

WebMD Healthy Shopping List

www.webmd.com/diet/printable/healthy-grocery-shopping-list

The WebMD shopping list is one of the best out there for consumers. It groups together foods with specific health points, for example, foods rich in omega-3 fatty acids, foods that contain plant sterols, foods high in fiber, foods high in potassium, and foods best to purchase organic. This list is also great because it gives some explanations for why you actually need these specific foods (e.g., high-fiber foods add bulk to your meal), is short and simple, easy to read, and great for people of any age.

The Ultimate Grocery List

www.grocerylists.org/ultimatest/

This is the lengthiest premade grocery list available. Not only does it cover the basics (vegetables, fruits, grains, and so on), but it also goes into cleaning products, office supplies, kitchen accessories, baby necessities, pet needs, personal hygiene products, and more. No insight on nutritional quality, though, and many unhealthy foods are listed (such as bacon, candy, and heavy cream). Choose wisely.

Thumbs Up! Healthy Eating

info@health-productions.com
2009 Health Production, LLC
P.O. Box 417
Milton, MA 02186

This booklet is chock full of colorful photographs providing strategies for building healthy meals and snacks. Tips are given to help you navigate each aisle of the supermarket including glossy shots of food labels and many brand-name products.

Appendixes

Conversion Tables/Equivalents

g = grams 1 gram =
1,000 mg
1 cup = 8 ounces
1 cup = 16 tablespoons

3 teaspoons = 1 tablespoon
28 grams (you can round it off to 30 to make calculations easier) = 1 ounce

Glossary of Nutrient Claims and Descriptors

Term	Description
Calorie-free	Less than 5 calories per serving.
Cholesterol-free	Less than 2 mg cholesterol and 2 grams or less saturated fat per serving.
Enriched or fortified	Has been nutritionally altered so that one serving provides at least 10 percent more of the Daily Value of a nutrient than the regular version.
Extra-lean	Less than 5 grams fat, 2 of which can be saturated, and 95 mg of cholesterol per serving and per 100 grams.
Fat-free	Less than 0.5 gram of fat per serving.
Free	"Without," "no," or "zero" are all synonyms.
Fresh	Generally used on food in its raw state. It cannot be used on food that has been frozen or cooked, or on food that contains preservatives.
Fresh-frozen	Foods that have been quickly frozen while still fresh.
Good source	One serving provides 10 to 19 percent of the Daily Value for a particular nutrient.
Good source of fiber	Contains 10 to 19 percent of the Daily Value for fiber (2.5 to 4.75 grams) per serving. If a food is not "low-fat," it must declare the level of total fat per serving and refer to the nutrition panel when a fiber claim is mentioned.
High	One serving provides at least 20 percent or more of the Daily Value for a particular nutrient.
High-fiber	Contains 20 percent or more of the Daily Value for fiber (at least 5 grams) per serving. If a food is not "low-fat," it must declare the level of total fat per serving and refer to the Nutrition Facts Panel when a fiber claim is made.
Lean	Less than 10 grams fat, 4 of which can be saturated, and 95 mg cholesterol per serving and per 100 grams.
Light	1) At least one-third fewer calories per serving than a comparison food;
	2) contains no more than half the fat per serving of a comparison food (if a food derives 50 percent or more of its calories from fat, the reduction must be at least 50 percent of the fat);
	3) contains at least 50 percent less sodium per serving than a comparison food; or
	4) can refer to texture and/or color, if clearly explained; for example, light brown sugar.
Low	"Little," "few," or "low source of" may be used in place of "low."
Low-calorie	40 calories or less per serving.
Low-cholesterol	20 mg or less cholesterol and 2 grams or less saturated fat per serving.
Low-fat	3 grams or less fat per serving.
Low saturated fat	1 gram or less saturated fat per serving and 15 percent or less calories from fat.
Low-sodium	140 mg or less sodium per serving.
More	One serving contains at least 10 percent more of the Daily Value of a nutrient than the regular version.
Percent fat-free	A claim made on a low-fat or fat-free product that accurately reflects the amount of fat present in 100 grams of food; a food with 3 grams of fat per 100 grams would be 97 percent fat-free.

Reduced	A nutritionally altered product that must contain 25 percent less of a nutrient or of calories than the regular version.
Salt- or sodium-free	Less than 5 mg per serving.
Sugar-free	Less than 0.5 gram of sugars per serving.
Unsalted	Has no salt added during processing. To use this term, the product must normally be processed with salt and the label must note that the food is not a sodium-free food if it does not meet the requirements for "sodium-free."
Very–low sodium	Less than 35 mg or less sodium per serving.

Food Additives and Preservatives

Just because a food contains an additive or a preservative doesn't necessarily mean that it is a food you should avoid. The Center for Science in the Public Interest (CSPI) has provided a detailed description of common food additives that range from being an important part of our daily food supply to those that we don't want anywhere near our plates. The following is a summary of their findings; they can be viewed in their entirety at www.cspinet.org.

Safety Summary

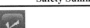 SAFE	CUT BACK	CAUTION	AVOID
These appear to be safe, though a few people may be allergic to any additive.	Not toxic, but large amounts may be unsafe or promote bad nutrition.	These additives may pose a risk and need to be better tested. Try to avoid them.	These additives are unsafe in the amounts consumed or are very poorly tested.

Alginate	Caffeine	Artificial colorings: Red No. 2, Red No. 40	Acesulfame potassium
Alpha-tocopherol (vitamin E)	Corn syrup	Brominated vegetable oil (BVO)	Artificial colorings: Blue No. 1, Blue No. 2, Green No. 3, Red No. 3, Yellow No. 6
Ascorbic acid (vitamin C)	Dextrose (corn sugar, glucose)	Butylated hydroxytoluene (BHT)	
Beta-carotene	Fructose	Diacetyl	Aspartame (NutraSweet)
Calcium propionate	High-fructose corn syrup	Heptyl paraben	Butylated hydroxyanisole (BHA)
Calcium stearoyl lactylate	Hydrogenated starch hydrolysate	Quinine	Cyclamate
Carrageenan	Invert sugar	Stevia	(not legal in the United States)
Citric acid	Lactitol		Hydrogenated vegetable oil
Diacylglycerol	Maltitol		Olestra (Olean)
EDTA	Mannitol		Partially hydrogenated vegetable oil
Erythorbic acid	Polydextrose		
Ferrous gluconate	Salatrim		Potassium bromate
Fumaric acid	Salt		Propyl gallate Saccharin
Gelatin	Sorbitol		Sodium nitrate
Glycerin (glycerol)	Sugar		Sodium nitrite
Gums: arabic, furcellaran, ghatti, guar, karaya, locust bean, xanthan	Tagatose		
High-maltose corn syrup	Xylitol		
Inulin			
Lactic acid			
Lecithin			
Maltodextrin			
Mono- and diglycerides Neotame			
Oat fiber, wheat fiber			
Oligofructose			
Phosphate salts			
Phosphoric acid			
Phytosterols and phytostanols			
Polysorbate 60, 65, 80			
Potassium sorbate			
Propylene glycol alginate			
Sodium ascorbate			
Sodium carboxymethylcellulose			

CERTAIN PEOPLE SHOULD AVOID

May cause allergic reactions or other problems. Artificial coloring:
Yellow No. 5
Artificial and natural flavoring
Benzoic acid
Caffeine
Carmine
Cochineal
Casein
Gum tragacanth
HVP (hydrolyzed vegetable protein)
Lactose
MSG (monosodium glutamate)
Mycoprotein
Quinine
Sodium benzoate

(CMC) Sodium citrate Sodium propionate Sodium stearoyl lactylate Sorbic acid Sorbitan monostearate Starch and modified starch Sucralose Thiamine mononitrate Triacetin (glycerol triacetate) Vanillin, ethyl vanillin Vegetable oil sterol esters		Sodium bisulfite Sodium caseinate Sulfites Sulfur dioxide	

Thanks so much for coming shopping with me and for reading *Read It Before You Eat It.*

It would be great to continue the conversation on social media so let's connect!

Follow Bonnie Taub-Dix, RDN:

www.BetterThanDieting.com

Instagram: @bonnietaubdix

@BTDmedia

Facebook: @Bonnietaubdix.rdn

Twitter: @eatsmartbd

Pinterest: Bonnietaubdix

Join the BetterThanDieting Community: bit.ly/fCeEuT

Made in the USA
Columbia, SC
13 December 2022

73684021R00100